121 W[...] TO LIVE 121 YEARS ...AND MORE!

Prescriptions for Longevity

Ronald Klatz, M.D., D.O.
President, American Academy of Anti-Aging Medicine

Robert Goldman, M.D., Ph.D., D.O., F.A.A.S.P.
President Emeritus, National Academy of Sports Medicine
Chairman, American Academy of Anti-Aging Medicine

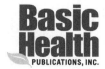

Basic Health
PUBLICATIONS, INC.

The information contained in this book is based upon the research and personal and professional experiences of the authors. It is not intended as a substitute for consulting with your physician or other healthcare provider. Any attempt to diagnose and treat an illness should be done under the direction of a healthcare professional.

The publisher does not advocate the use of any particular healthcare protocol but believes the information in this book should be available to the public. The publisher and authors are not responsible for any adverse effects or consequences resulting from the use of the suggestions, preparations, or procedures discussed in this book. Should the reader have any questions concerning the appropriateness of any procedures or preparation mentioned, the authors and the publisher strongly suggest consulting a professional healthcare advisor.

Basic Health Publications, Inc.
28812 Top of the World Drive
Laguna Beach, CA 92651
949-715-7327 • www.basichealthpub.com

Library of Congress Cataloging-in-Publication Data

Klatz, Ronald.
    121 ways to live 121 years—and more! : prescriptions for longevity /
Ronald Klatz, Robert Goldman.
        p. cm.
    Originally published: Chicago : American Academy of Anti-Aging Medicine,
c2005.
        ISBN-10: 1-59120-197-7
        ISBN-13: 978-1-59120-197-7
    1. Longevity—Popular works. I. Goldman, Bob. II. Title.

    RA776.75.K525   2006
    613'.0438—dc22

                                                                    2006025179

Researcher and Editor: Catherine Cebula
In-house Editor: Carol Rosenberg
Typesetting and Book Design: Gary A. Rosenberg
Cover Design: Mike Stromberg

Printed in the United States of America

10   9   8   7   6   5   4   3   2   1

Contents

Introduction

*To know how to grow old is the master work
of wisdom, and one of the most difficult
chapters in the great art of living.*
—Henri Frederic Amiel, Swiss philosopher

Webster's New World Dictionary defines "aging" as "the process of growing old or showing signs of growing old." While this definition may have sufficed for the nineteenth century when Mr. Webster was alive, new medical discoveries and biotechnological advancements have made the Webster definition of "aging" outmoded.

Today, aging may be segregated into two very different concepts—chronological age and biological age. In celebrating a birthday, we commemorate our advancing chronological age. The performance of our body systems—from mental function to sexual performance to physical strength—reflects our biological age. Most of us know at least one person whose driver's license says he or she is over seventy, but we observe that person carrying on in his or her daily life with the vibrancy expected of someone twenty to thirty years younger. Conversely, you may know someone with the chronological age of forty who fails to go about life with the energy expected for that age. Scientists now agree that it is biological age that makes a difference in how long, and how well, we live our lives.

Today, scientists know much more about the deterioration and vulnerability to disease that contribute to biological aging. The contemporary approach to aging submits that the disabilities and diseases associated with what we consider as "normal aging" are caused by physiological dysfunctions that, in many cases, respond to medical treatment. As a result, the human life span can be increased while the quality of life is maintained or improved. In short, biological aging can be beneficially impacted, and aging is not inevitable.

This contemporary approach to aging, known as anti-aging medicine, is a clinical specialty practiced by more than 30,000 physicians in eighty-five countries worldwide (as of 2006). The world's fastest growing new medical specialty, anti-aging medicine applies advanced scientific and medical technologies for the early detection, prevention, treatment, and reversal of age-related dysfunction, disorders, and diseases. The goal of anti-aging medicine is not to merely prolong the total years of an individual's life, but to ensure that those years are enjoyed in a productive and vital fashion. Anti-aging medicine is based on principles of sound and responsible medical care that are consistent with those applied in other preventive health specialties.

In addition, anti-aging medicine integrates high-tech diagnostic and treatment biomedical technologies to achieve the very earliest detection and most aggressive care of disease. CT, ultrasound, and PET scans; stem-cell research; genetic engineering; and nanotechnology are integral components of this fast-growing specialty of preventive medicine.

Learning By Imitation—The Longest-Lived Animals

- Oldest tortoise: 188 years

- Oldest fish (eel): 88 years

- Oldest primate (chimpanzee): 71 years

- Oldest alligator: 66 years

- Oldest goldfish: 43 years

- Oldest snake (boa): 40 years, 3 months, 2 weeks

If these and other animals can enjoy increased healthy life spans, then with simple, practical lifestyle and habit changes people can, too.

Visit the World Health Network at www.worldhealth.net. Sign up for the FREE BioTech e-Newsletter to learn how to live longer and better, starting today!

THE ESSENTIAL RULES OF ANTI-AGING MEDICINE

1. Don't get sick. 2. Don't get old. 3. Don't die.

Corollaries to Follow

• **Pick your physician carefully**—The U.S. Department of Health and Human Services reported that physicians cause 120,000 or more accidental deaths a year in the United States. Averaging that across the approximate number of physicians in the United States (700,000), the rate of accidental deaths per physician is 0.171. Comparing with a rate of accidental deaths per gun owner of 0.000188, doctors are statistically 9,000 times more dangerous than guns!

It is preferable to choose a physician who will serve as your health partner and empower you with the knowledge necessary to make educated medical decisions. Board-certified anti-aging physicians serve well in this role: find one in your geographical area by using the interactive directory at the World Health Network, www.worldhealth.net.

• **Stay out of the hospital**—Researchers from the University College London reported in the *British Medical Journal* that you have a 10 percent chance of being harmed during a stay at the hospital. The team also found that about 50 percent of these cases could have been prevented by hospital staff. One-third of the mishaps caused "moderate or greater impairment," and in 19 percent of the cases, the mistake was irreversible. A full 6 percent of the mistakes were deadly. In 2005, the U.S. nonprofit organization Consumers Union reported that one out of every twenty people admitted to a hospital acquires an infection during their stay. That translates into 2 million people—of which 90,000 die each year, more than the number of deaths from auto accidents and homicides combined.

• **The bottom line**—You must learn enough, and keep learning, about how to keep yourself healthy. Be your own health advocate and control your health destiny. Don't entrust your wellness to someone other than yourself.

Anti-aging medicine represents the dawning of an exciting new era in medicine, one that will result with longevity intervention orders of magnitude greater than any other advancements made in medicine to date. Enjoy a future of boundless health and vitality by implementing anti-aging approaches to help you feel, look, and perform better today.

Start by enjoying *121 Ways to Live to 121 Years . . . and More!*, and make this your handbook for living a long and healthy life. As cofounders of the anti-aging medical movement, we have combined our fifty years of medical know-how in this book to provide hundreds of practical tips that you can implement today to help you live a satisfying and productive tomorrow. Notice that we share with you the science behind each tip, to empower you with knowledge so you can act as your own health advocate.

A FEW REMINDERS

Dosing of nutraceuticals can be highly variable. Proper dosing is based on parameters that include sex, age, and whether a person is well or ill (and, if ill, whether it is a chronic or acute condition). Additionally, efficiency of absorption of a particular type of product and the quality of its individual ingredients are two major considerations for choosing appropriate specific agents for an individual's medical situation. Furthermore, anyone with cancer should consult their physician or oncologist prior to beginning, or continuing, any hormone therapy program.

Please be mindful that just because a product is natural doesn't mean it's safe for everyone. A small portion of the general population may react adversely to components in nutraceuticals (especially botanical products). Make your physician aware of any and all interventions you use regularly, and seek medical consultation before starting any others.

If you are interested in learning more about the suggestions, preparations, or procedures mentioned in this book, we urge you to consult a knowledgeable physician or health practitioner, preferably one who is board certified in anti-aging medicine. You may find one by using the interactive directory at the educational website of the American Academy of Anti-Aging Medicine (A4M), www.worldhealth.net, or you may call the A4M's international headquarters in Chicago, Illinois, at 773-528-4333.

How to Use This Book

"For the great benefits of our being—our life, health, and reason, we look upon ourselves."
—MARCUS ANNAEUS SENECA, ROMAN WRITER

In *121 Ways to Live to 121 Years . . . and More!*, we cover thirteen categories of topics that relate to improving the healthy human life span, and include hundreds of individual tips on a wide variety of subjects. At the top of each page, you'll see a small icon. Icons represent the following topics:

 Anti-Aging Intelligence—presenting important concepts in anti-aging medicine

 Beat the Leading Causes of Death—reducing your risk of developing heart disease, cancer, stroke, diabetes, and Alzheimer's disease

 Beauty—looking great at any age

 Body Fitness—maintaining your peak physical performance

 Brain Fitness—optimizing your mental acuity

Detoxification and Purification—reducing the toxic load that may contribute to disease

 Food Facts—describing the role of foods in disease prevention

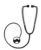 **Lifestyle Basics**—making simple changes in daily habits to live longer and better

 Preparedness—taking charge to be ready for a variety of emergency situations

 Sex—enjoying your partner's company safely

 Sleep—getting the best rest of your life

 Stress Reduction—lowering the taxing burden of everyday life

 What's Eating You—maximizing your immune system to ward off disease

As we explain in the Introduction, each of us needs to be our own health advocate and control our health destiny. We must learn enough, and keep learning, about how to keep ourselves healthy. Self-reliance is the key to our health, happiness, and well-being.

1

Knowledge Is Power

Medical and scientific knowledge doubles every three and a half years or less. Within sixteen years, we will know thirty-two times more about how and why we age, and how to treat it. Become educated, and stay atop of the newest breakthroughs, and you too can live a long and healthy life. Assemble a handy list of reliable resources. We recommend:

- The World Health Network at www.worldhealth.net. With more than 14 million hits a month, the World Health Network, the educational website of the American Academy of Anti-Aging Medicine (A4M), features an extensive library of articles relating to longevity.

- While at the World Health Network website, sign up for the free BioTech e-Newsletter. Delivered electronically to your e-mail inbox, the newsletter highlights the latest advancements in anti-aging medical research and clinical science.

> *"The only good is knowledge,*
> *and the only evil ignorance."*
>
> —LAËRTIUS DIOGENES,
> BIOGRAPHER OF GREEK PHILOSOPHERS

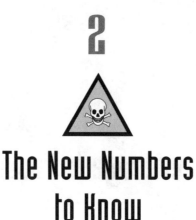

2

The New Numbers to Know

It's not enough to know your cholesterol level. While cholesterol is the molecule responsible for causing fatty buildups inside arteries, scientists now suspect that it is only part of the portrait of heart disease. Inflammation, which can weaken blood vessels and cause cholesterol plaques to loosen and create blockages, is the new marker. Insist that your doctor test your C-reactive protein (CRP), which should be at or below 8 micrograms/milliliter (anti-aging physicians would prefer it to be half that or lower). In addition, in women, elevated white blood cell counts may predict heart disease, reports a 2005 Women's Health Initiative study. Levels at the upper end of normal (6.7 billion white blood cells per liter of blood) may double a woman's risk of heart attack.

> *"Coronary heart disease is now the leading cause of death worldwide. It is on the rise and has become a true pandemic that respects no borders."*
> —WORLD HEALTH ORGANIZATION

Meats and Sweets
Are Not Healthy Treats

Dietary factors, second only to tobacco as a preventable cause of cancer, account for about 30 percent of all cancers in Western countries and approximately 20 percent in developing countries. Announcing findings in 2005 of its twenty-year-long study tracking 150,000 Americans, the American Cancer Society found that men and women who ate the most amounts of red meat (compared with those who ate more poultry, fish, and non-meats) had a 53 percent higher risk of distal colon cancer. Also in 2005, a study by Johns Hopkins Bloomberg School of Health, in which 1 million Koreans were tracked for ten years, reported that high sugar consumption could be a risk factor in developing several types of cancer. These researchers suggest that glucose intolerance may be one way that obesity increases cancer risk and that rising obesity rates may increase future cancer rates.

"More than 11 million people are diagnosed with cancer every year. It is estimated that there will be 16 million new cases every year by 2020."
—WORLD HEALTH ORGANIZATION

4

Smoke Out Stroke

Cigarette smoking is a major, preventable risk factor for stroke. The nicotine and carbon monoxide in tobacco smoke reduce the amount of oxygen in your blood. They also damage the walls of blood vessels, making clots more likely to form.

When smokers quit, the body begins a series of changes. According to the American Lung Association: At twenty minutes after quitting, blood pressure decreases and pulse rate drops. At eight hours after quitting, carbon monoxide levels in your blood drop to normal, and oxygen levels increase to normal. In as little as twenty-four hours, you cut your risk of having a stroke or heart attack.

If you are unable to quit smoking, there are some nutritional supplements that may help protect your body's cells from the damage caused by smoking. Find out more by visiting the World Health Network at www.worldhealth.net, the website of the A4M.

5

Packing on the Pounds Increases Diabetes Risk

A 2005 study by researchers at University of Newcastle upon Tyne in the United Kingdom found that men and women with a higher body fat and higher waist-hip ratio are more likely to have increased insulin resistance, a risk marker for type 2 diabetes. Childhood factors, such as birth weight and nutrition, were found to have little impact on the risk of developing diabetes, discounting the notion that poor health in later life can result from earlier experiences.

*"Recently compiled data show that approximately
150 million people have diabetes mellitus worldwide, and
that this number may well double by the year 2025."*
—WORLD HEALTH ORGANIZATION

6

Know the Signs

Worldwide, a substantial number of men and women who have coronary artery disease die within twenty-eight days after experiencing symptoms; of these, two-thirds die before reaching a hospital. It is critical that everyone recognizes the warning signs of a heart attack, which may include:

- **Chest discomfort**—Most heart attacks involve discomfort in the center of the chest that lasts for more than a few minutes, or goes away and comes back. The discomfort can feel like uncomfortable pressure, squeezing, fullness, or pain.

- **Discomfort in other areas of the upper body**—Can include pain or discomfort in one or both arms, the back, neck, jaw, or stomach.

- **Shortness of breath**—Often comes along with chest discomfort. But it also can occur before chest discomfort.

- **Other symptoms**—May include breaking out in a cold sweat, nausea, or light-headedness.

If you think you are experiencing heart attack symptoms, do not delay. Minutes matter! Call 911 immediately. While waiting for an ambulance, chew one adult-strength (325 mg) aspirin tablet: Aspirin reduces the risk of death by up to 23 percent if administered when a heart attack is suspected, and for thirty days thereafter. The use of aspirin as first aid for a heart attack could potentially save 10,000 lives each year in the United States alone.

> *"3.8 million men and 3.4 million women worldwide die each year from coronary heart disease."*
>
> —WORLD HEALTH ORGANIZATION

7

Exercise the Body to Keep the Brain Fit

A 2005 Finnish study revealed that middle-aged men and women who exercise at least twice a week and eat a healthy diet can reduce their risk of developing Alzheimer's disease (AD) by 50 percent in old age. Previous studies have shown that people with high blood pressure, high cholesterol, and who are overweight or obese could have a greater risk of AD than those with a more active, healthy lifestyle.

"Worldwide, 37 million people live with dementia, with Alzheimer's disease causing the majority of cases."
—WORLD HEALTH ORGANIZATION

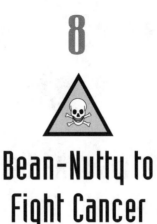

Bean-Nutty to Fight Cancer

A compound found in everyday foods can slow the development of cancerous tumors. A 2005 study conducted by scientists at the University College of London's Sackler Institute found that inositol pentakisphosphate can inhibit an enzyme that is necessary for tumors to grow.

Each day, try to eat foods rich in inositol pentakisphosphate: 1 cup (226 g) of beans (such as lentils and peas), $\frac{1}{2}$ cup (113 g) of nuts (almonds and hazelnuts [filberts] are also good sources of vitamin E—see Tip 31) and 6 ounces (170 g) of whole-wheat cereals (for the wheat bran).

> *"In the U.S., cancer has surpassed heart disease as the leading cause of death for those 85 years of age and under."*
> —U.S. NATIONAL CENTER FOR HEALTH STATISTICS

9

DASH for Life

Treating hypertension (high blood pressure) can reduce the risk of a stroke by up to 40 percent, reports the World Health Organization. High blood pressure (generally, 140/90 mm Hg or higher; however, anti-aging physicians aim for readings less than 120/80) is the most important risk factor for stroke.

The U.S. government's Dietary Approaches to Stop Hypertension (DASH) diet can help, providing menus low in salt and calories and high in nutrients. Consume a variety of nuts, seeds, and beans; watch your intake of meats, poultry, and fish; and expand your repertoire of vegetables. Go easy on processed foods, salty snacks, and cured meats.

Go to www.nhlbi.nih.gov/health, the website of the U.S. National Heart, Lung, and Blood Institute, look under "Recipe Collections," and select "The DASH Eating Plan."

10

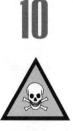

Diabetics at Increased Risk of Heart Disease

Diabetics with a particular form of a blood protein, called hapto-globin, have as much as a 500 percent increased risk of developing heart disease. In a study by Technion–Israel Institute of Technology, researchers found that vitamin E supplements (both natural and mixed forms) helped diabetic men and women who have the 2-2 form of haptoglobin to reduce their risk of heart attacks and dying from diabetes-related heart disease. It is estimated that 40 percent of diabetics have this blood protein variant, so as many as two of every five diabetics could benefit from taking vitamin E supplements.

"Heart disease accounts for approximately 50 percent of all deaths among people with diabetes in industrialized countries."
—WORLD HEALTH ORGANIZATION

11

Attitude & Alzheimer's

In 2005, researchers from Rush University Medical Center reported that people who tend to worry or feel stressed out may be more likely to develop Alzheimer's disease (AD) later in life. The team surveyed 1,064 men and women ages sixty-five and over about their tendencies toward worry and stress. Those who appeared prone to feeling distressed were twice as likely to develop AD within the three- to six-year follow-up timeframe.

> *"A man's doubts and fears*
> *are his worst enemies."*
>
> —WILLIAM WRIGLEY, JR.,
> GRANDSON OF U.S. CHEWING GUM INDUSTRIALIST

12

Eat Your Heart Out

Men and women with heart disease can reduce their likelihood of dying by up to 30 percent by enjoying a Mediterranean-style diet, reports a 2005 study coauthored by researchers at Harvard University and Athens Medical School in Greece.

Opt for colorful vegetables (such as lycopene-rich tomatoes) and fruits (like antioxidant-rich red and purple grapes), cut your consumption of meat and dairy products, and boost your consumption of monounsaturated and polyunsaturated fatty acids, such as olive oil and omega-3–rich foods like fish, soy, grains, and leafy green vegetables.

"While genetic factors play a part, 80 to 90 percent of people dying from coronary heart disease have one or more major risk factors that are influenced by lifestyle."

—WORLD HEALTH ORGANIZATION

13

Prevent Prostate Problems

Prostate cancer is a major cause of death among men. It has claimed the lives of 56,000 European men (in 1998), along with 29,900 American men (in 2004). To date, there have been no obvious preventive strategies; however, in 2005 scientists from the Northern California Cancer Center proposed that vitamin D may cut prostate cancer risk. The researchers found that in men with certain gene variants, high sun exposure reduced prostate cancer risk by as much as 65 percent. Previous research has shown that the prostate uses vitamin D, which the body manufactures from exposure to sunlight, to promote the normal growth of prostate cells and to inhibit the invasiveness and spread of prostate cancer cells to other parts of the body.

The scientists propose that men may benefit by increasing vitamin D intake from diet and supplements (whereas excessive exposure to sunlight may result with the negative effect of sun-induced skin cancer). Foods rich in vitamin D include egg yolks, liver, and cod-liver oil. Margarine and cereals are often fortified with this nutrient as well.

Learn more about reducing your cancer risk factors by visiting the World Health Network at www.worldhealth.net, the website of the A4M.

14

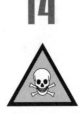

Fish Around and Cut Your Stroke Risk

Having tracked the diet of 4,775 adults for twelve years, in 2005 Harvard University scientists revealed findings on the association between different types of fish meals and the risk of stroke in men and women ages sixty-five and older. They found that eating broiled or baked fish one to four times per week lowered stroke risk by 28 percent, and dining on the same for five or more times per week reduced the risk by 32 percent. By comparison, fried fish and fish sandwich consumption was associated with a 37 percent increased risk of stroke.

> *"Several foods and nutrients have been linked to the risk of stroke; therefore, dietary modification may be an important way to reduce the risk of stroke."*
>
> —*STROKE* JOURNAL REPORT

15

Delaying Diabetes

New data models derived from the Diabetes Prevention Project by the University of Michigan Health System show that men and women who walked briskly for thirty minutes five days a week lowered their fat and calorie intake, achieved a weight-reduction goal of 7 percent of body weight over a three-year period, and were able to cut their risk of developing type 2 diabetes by 58 percent.

> *"A person with diabetes incurs medical costs that are two to five times higher than those of a person without diabetes. This is due to more frequent medical visits, purchase of supplies and medication, and the higher likelihood of being admitted to a hospital."*
>
> —INTERNATIONAL DIABETES FEDERATION

16

Brush and Floss to Save Your Brain

In a 2005 study by University of South Carolina, periodontal disease, marked by missing teeth and gum disease, at an early age correlated to an increased risk of Alzheimer's disease (AD).

Researchers tracked the lifestyles of more than 100 pairs of identical twins, each of which included one twin who developed dementia and one who did not. Twins who had severe periodontal disease before the age of thirty-five had a five-fold increased risk in developing AD. This study is considered further evidence that chronic inflammation in the body can damage the brain.

Find out more about Alzheimer's disease by visiting the World Health Network at www.worldhealth.net, the website of the A4M.

17

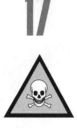

Fit In When You're Young

Young men and women who are fit—guys who are able to complete ten to twelve minutes of treadmill exercise, gals who are able to complete six to nine minutes of the same—are half as likely to develop high blood pressure, a major risk factor for heart disease, reports a study sponsored by the U.S. National Heart, Lung, and Blood Institute. As side benefits, fit youths cut their risk of developing diabetes by 50 percent and tend to gain far less weight (compared with their less-fit counterparts) over the long term.

> *"Heart disease is a major public-health problem that is responsible for one third of annual global deaths and one tenth of the global disease burden. [The] challenge [is] to provide a comprehensive strategy to promote heart health among children and teenagers."*
> —PAN AMERICAN HEALTH ORGANIZATION

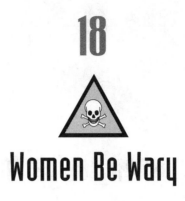

18

Women Be Wary

While the Pap smear is a test doctors routinely conduct to check women for cervical cancer, this test may not find abnormal cells in the cervix until cancer has already developed. A new test, the human papilloma virus (HPV) test, detects elevated levels of the infectious pathogen that is the cause of nearly all cases of cervical cancer.

HPV is harbored by an estimated 80 percent of sexually active adults, but the majority of infections clear up without incident. If you are younger than thirty, experts now recommended that you have the HPV test if your Pap smear test is unclear. If you are thirty or older, experts recommend you have the HPV test at the same time as your Pap test. A new vaccine for cervical cancer is now available. The vaccine targets HPV types 16 and 18, thought to cause 70 percent of cervical cancers, and HPV types 6 and 11, associated with 90 percent of genital warts cases.

Find out more about sexually transmitted diseases by visiting the World Health Network at www.worldhealth.net, the website of the A4M.

19

Exercise Melts Pounds, Wards Off Diabetes

Physical activity can help people with diabetes control their blood glucose, weight, and blood pressure, as well as raise their "good" cholesterol (HDL) and lower their "bad" cholesterol (LDL). It can also help prevent heart and blood flow problems, reducing the risk of heart disease and nerve damage, which are often problems for people with diabetes.

Generally, diabetics should engage in moderate-intensity physical activity for at least thirty minutes on five or more days of the week. Some examples of moderate-intensity physical activity are walking briskly, mowing the lawn, dancing, swimming, or bicycling.

If you are not accustomed to physical activity, you may want to start with a little exercise, and work your way up. As you become stronger, you can add a few extra minutes to your physical activity. Do some physical activity every day, rather than an extended period of activity once a week.

> *"Even moderate reduction in weight and only half an hour of walking each day reduced the incidence of diabetes by more than one half."*
>
> —WORLD HEALTH ORGANIZATION

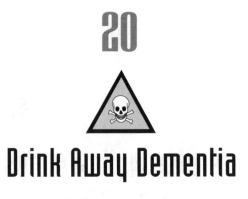

20

Drink Away Dementia

A Japanese study reported that compounds found in wine may inhibit Alzheimer's disease (AD). Small pre-proteins (peptides) found in red and white wines inhibit an enzyme implicated in the production and accumulation of amyloid plaques, which deposit in the brain and cause memory loss.

The greatest concentrations of these AD-busting peptides are found in Merlot (California), Sauvignon Blanc (Bordeaux), and Pinot Noir wines, and was also detected in the juice and pulp parts of grapes. Teetotalers may wish to try the nutritional supplement, resveratrol, the active therapeutic ingredient in wine.

> *"Wine is the most healthful*
> *and most hygienic of beverages."*
> —LOUIS PASTEUR,
> FRENCH MICROBIOLOGIST AND CHEMIST

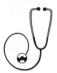

Butt Out Sooner, Live Longer

A fifty-year long tobacco study of smoking and death in the United Kingdom found that on average, cigarette smokers die ten years younger than nonsmokers. But stopping at age fifty cuts the risk in half, and stopping at age thirty avoids almost all of it. Similar findings were published in a 2005 study of Americans. Researchers from the University of Minnesota School of Public Health tracked 5,887 middle-aged smokers with mild lung disease for fourteen years. Those who were able to quit smoking experienced a 46 percent lower death rate, and those who simply tried to quit also experienced lower death rates (compared with those who continued to smoke). Quitting smoking also reduces your risk of stroke (see Tip 4).

> *"Cigarette smoke contains about 4,000 chemicals including over 60 carcinogens (cancer-causing agents). In addition, many of these substances, such as carbon monoxide, tar, arsenic, and lead, are poisonous and toxic to the human body."*
> —U.S. NATIONAL CANCER INSTITUTE

22

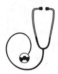

Multivitamin + Multimineral = Multibeneficial

Researchers from Memorial University in Newfoundland found that a dietary supplement containing eighteen vitamins, minerals, and trace elements helped healthy men and women ages sixty-five and over to improve their short-term memory, problem-solving ability, abstract thinking, and attention span. The supplement also improved immunity, reducing the rate of infection-related illness by more than 50 percent (compared with those who did not take it).

This study demonstrates that people who take a daily multivitamin, multimineral supplement enhance their ability to live independently and without major disability. The researchers also calculated that for every one U.S. dollar spent on the supplement, twenty-eight U.S. dollars could be saved in healthcare costs by preventing or delaying illness and functional decline.

Visit the World Health Network at www.worldhealth.net, the website of the A4M, to learn the latest on anti-aging therapeutics that may extend and enhance your healthy life span.

23

Lower Pressure with Potatoes

Potatoes are among the foods richest in potassium, a mineral that fights high blood pressure. One baked potato with skin contains 903 mg of potassium, nearly one-third of the recommended daily value. And, in 2005, researchers from the Institute of Food Research in the United Kingdom found that the potato contains natural compounds known as kukoamines, which in an herbal remedy (*Lycium chinense*) are associated with blood-pressure-reducing properties.

> *"It's easy to halve the potato*
> *where there's love."*
> —IRISH PROVERB

24

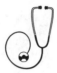

Careful Fun in the Sun

Sunburn most commonly happens between 10 A.M. and 3 P.M., when ultraviolet (UV) rays are at their strongest. Wear sunscreen with a sun protection factor (SPF) of 15 or greater, when you expect to be out in the sun for more than fifteen minutes (a little sun is good for you, see Tip 45). Ladies will also benefit by wearing facial makeup containing SPF.

Sunlight can damage the sensitive cells of the macula (the central part of the eye that is responsible for most of our vision), so be sure to wear sunglasses (pick shades that block 99 percent of UV-A and UV-B rays), and wear a wide-brimmed hat.

"Excessive solar ultraviolet radiation increases the risk of all types of cancer of the skin. Avoiding excessive exposure, use of sunscreen and protective clothing are effective preventive measures."
—WORLD HEALTH ORGANIZATION

25

Defend Against Atomic Pickpockets: Vitamin A

Antioxidant supplements (vitamin A, C, E, and selenium) protect cells by neutralizing free radicals, atomic fragments that cause cellular destruction and produce metabolic waste.

Numerous studies point to the value of vitamin A in boosting immunity, as it enhances Th2 (T-helper cell type 2) mediated immune responses, necessary for fighting bacterial and parasitic infections. In addition, several studies have shown that vitamin A is a potent stimulator of growth hormone production.

Therapeutic daily dose: 7,000–10,000 IU. People over age sixty-five, those with liver disease, and women who are or could become pregnant should speak with their doctors, as limited vitamin A intake may be appropriate.

Sign up at the World Health Network, www.worldhealth.net, the website of the A4M, for the FREE BioTech e-Newsletter, which shares insights on how you can live longer and better.

26

Say "No" to Nitrites

Preserved and cured meats such as bacon, sausage, and deli meats are the largest source of nitrites in our diet. Nitrites cause the body to form nitrosamines, which are environmental oxidants and powerful carcinogens. Scientists have established a significant association between nitrosamines and stomach cancer.

> *"Tell me what you eat,*
> *and I will tell you what you are."*
> —JEAN ANTHELME BRILLAT-SAVARIN,
> FRENCH EPICURE AND GASTRONOME

27

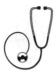

Happiness Helps Health

A 2005 study of middle-aged men and women living in the United Kingdom found that people who are happier in their daily lives have healthier levels of key body chemicals than those who have few positive feelings. This University College London study is the first to link everyday happiness with lower levels of the stress hormone, cortisol, and reduced levels of the blood protein fibrinogen, which causes red blood cells to clot and may contribute to coronary heart disease.

"Not only is there a right to be happy,
there is a duty to be happy. So much sadness
exists in the world that we are all under obligation
to contribute as much joy as lies within our powers."
—JOHN SUTHERLAND POWELL,
AUTHOR OF *HAPPINESS IS AN INSIDE JOB*

28

Defend Against Atomic
Pickpockets: Vitamin C

Antioxidant supplements (vitamin A, C, E, and selenium) protect cells by neutralizing free radicals, atomic fragments that cause cellular destruction and produce metabolic waste.

Vitamin C raises "good" cholesterol (HDL), and prevents "bad" cholesterol (LDL) from oxidation, which subsequently prevents the buildup of athlerosclerotic plaques on the blood vessel wall that contributes to cardiovascular disease. In a study by University of California–Los Angeles School of Health, men who took vitamin C daily had a 45 percent lower risk of heart attack than men whose intake was less than the U.S. RDA. Vitamin C has also been found to lower the risk of stroke. In one study, men who had relatively low blood levels of vitamin C were 2.4 times more likely to have a stroke than men with the highest blood levels of the nutrient. In a separate study, women who took supplemental vitamin C over a ten-year period were 77 percent less likely to develop lens opacities, the beginning stage of cataracts (compared with women who didn't take supplementary vitamin C).

Therapeutic daily dose: 1,000–2,000 mg. Some medical conditions preclude vitamin C supplementation; check with your doctor.

Visit the World Health Network at www.worldhealth.net, the website of the A4M, to learn the latest on anti-aging therapeutics that may extend and enhance your healthy life span.

29

Eat for Long Life

Okinawa has the highest proportion of centenarians—men and women ages 100 years or older—in the world. Okinawans have 80 percent fewer heart attacks than Americans, and 75 percent fewer cancers, including breast cancer and cancer of the ovaries in women and prostate cancer in men.

A Johns Hopkins study of 600 Okinawan men and women attributes their longevity to a low-calorie diet that typically features:

- No fewer than seven servings of vegetables daily, featuring dark-green vegetables (rich in calcium)

- Seven or more daily servings of grains in the form of noodles, bread, and rice (many of them whole grains)

- Two to four servings of fruit a day

- Abundance of tofu and other forms of soy

- Three weekly servings of fish, rich in omega-3 fatty acids

- Alcohol in moderation (women: one drink a day; men: two drinks a day)

In short, the Okinawan diet is rich in complex carbohydrates and plant-based foods, and low in fat, compared with the average Western diet.

"Thou shalt eat to live, not live to eat."
—CICERO, ORATOR AND STATESMAN OF ANCIENT ROME

30

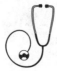

Look on the Bright Side of Life

Older adults with a bright outlook on the future live longer than those who have a dimmer view. A nine-year study conducted by Netherlands researchers found that men and women with the highest levels of optimism at the start of the study had the lowest death rates than those in the most pessimistic group. Considering all factors in total, the risk of death was 29 percent lower among highly optimistic men and women. In addition, the most optimistic study participants experienced 77 percent less likelihood of dying of a heart attack, stroke, or other cardiovascular cause (compared with the most pessimistic group).

"Why do some people always see beautiful skies and grass and lovely flowers and incredible human beings, while others are hard-pressed to find anything or any place that is beautiful?"

—LEO BUSCAGLIA, BEST-SELLING AUTHOR

31

Defend Against Atomic Pickpockets: Vitamin E

Antioxidant supplements (vitamin A, C, E, and selenium) protect cells by neutralizing free radicals, atomic fragments that cause cellular destruction and produce metabolic waste.

The Alpha Tocopherol-Beta Carotene Study, which involved more than 29,000 men, revealed that those who took vitamin E supplements were 32 percent less likely to develop prostate cancer and 41 percent less likely to die from the disease. In 2005, researchers involved in the Women's Health Study, the largest trial to date involving vitamin E supplementation, reported that natural alpha-tocopherol supplements significantly lowered the risk of death, especially by heart attack and stroke, and particularly in women over age sixty-five. A separate study found that consuming high dietary levels of vitamin E could lower the risk of developing Alzheimer's disease by as much as 70 percent.

Therapeutic daily dose: 400–1,200 IU. Choose only natural vitamin E supplements (mixed natural tocopherols), as natural forms are more potent and bioavailable than synthetic forms. Some medical conditions preclude vitamin E supplementation: check with your doctor.

Sign up at the World Health Network, www.worldhealth.net, the website of the A4M, for the FREE BioTech e-Newsletter, which shares insights on how you can live longer and better.

32

Head Off Headaches, Joint Pain, Heart Disease, and Cancer

A compound found in olive oil, called oleocanthal, has anti-inflammatory properties much like those associated with the painkiller ibuprofen, an NSAID (see Tip 40), found U.S. researchers in 2005.

Oleocanthal inhibits COX enzymes responsible for the inflammatory response implicated in headaches and joint pain. This study not only supports that regular consumption of olive oil might have some of the long-term health benefits of ibuprofen (that is, the minimization of joint swelling), but may help explain olive oil's widely reported health benefits such as in lowering the rates of heart disease and cancer in populations that consume it in large quantities (such as Mediterranean countries). The study authors conclude that "Our findings raise the possibility that long-term consumption of oleocanthal may help to protect against some diseases."

> *"He's the best physician that knows
> the worthlessness of most medicines."*
>
> —BENJAMIN FRANKLIN,
> AMERICAN STATESMAN AND INVENTOR

33

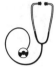

Keep Your Family Close, and Your Friends Closer

People with a close circle of friends may outlive those who merely have strong family ties. From the Australian Longitudinal Study of Aging, involving 1,477 men and women ages seventy and over, researchers from Flinders University in Australia determined in 2005 that greater networks of friends protected against death during a ten-year study period. Having a small circle of confidants, or a social network comprised solely of relatives, were far weaker contributors to longevity.

"Without friends, no one would choose to live, though he had all other goods."

—ARISTOTLE, GREEK PHILOSOPHER

34

Defend Against Atomic Pickpockets: Selenium

Antioxidant supplements (vitamin A, C, E, and selenium) protect cells by neutralizing free radicals, atomic fragments that cause cellular destruction and produce metabolic waste.

Selenium is an essential trace element, necessary for growth and protein synthesis. It helps to increase the effectiveness of vitamin E, another key antioxidant (see Tip 31). Selenium may help to prevent cardiovascular diseases by increasing levels of "good" cholesterol (HDL), lowering levels of "bad" cholesterol (LDL), and decreasing the "stickiness" of blood to reduce the risk of blood clots in arteries supplying the heart and brain.

Selenium has been shown to offer protection against a number of different types of cancer. Results of two five-year-long studies at Cornell University and the University of Arizona revealed that daily supplemental selenium cut the incidence of prostate cancer by 63 percent, colorectal tumors by 58 percent, and lung cancer by 46 percent. In these studies, all tolled, the death rate from cancer of people who took supplemental selenium was found to be 39 percent lower than that of the general population.

Therapeutic daily dose: 100–200 mcg.

Visit the World Health Network at www.worldhealth.net, the website of the A4M, to learn the latest on anti-aging therapeutics that may extend and enhance your healthy life span.

35

The Not-So-Killer Tomato

Tomatoes are rich in lycopene, an antioxidant nutrient that has been associated with heart health, and, in men, with prostate health. Enjoy fresh tomatoes from local growers when in season. Other times of the year, reach for processed tomatoes knowing that ketchup, tomato paste, and pasta sauces pack even more lycopenes because they are concentrated during the reduction process. Opt for low-sugar, low-salt varieties when choosing processed tomato products.

Sign up at the World Health Network, www.worldhealth.net, the website of the A4M, for the FREE BioTech e-Newsletter, which shares insights on how you can live longer and better.

36

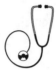

Water, the Elixir of Life

Water is a critical component of your optimal health program. A person can go many days, even weeks, without food—but deprived of water, life can end within three days. Water composes more than half our bodies, one-quarter of our bones, and one-third of our brains. It is present in every cell and tissue of the body, and every bodily function—from breathing to eating to thinking—is utterly dependent upon it.

Drink one 8-ounce (236-ml) glass of distilled water, with a pinch of sea salt (for electrolytes), every one to two hours that you are awake. You may need to drink more when you are physically active.

"Water is the only drink for a wise man."

—HENRY DAVID THOREAU, AMERICAN AUTHOR

37

Anti-Aging Aid:
Aspirin

Aspirin can lower a person's risk of death from any cause, even in men and women who are so inactive that their inactivity increases their risk of death. A daily low dose of aspirin (81 mg) can cut the risk of death in people known or thought to have heart disease by as much as 30 to 40 percent, by preventing platelet aggregation.

A review of nearly 300 studies into the benefits of aspirin has confirmed that low doses of the drug can dramatically reduce the risk of death from heart attack or stroke. People treated with aspirin or other anti-platelet drugs were 33 percent less likely to have a heart attack, 25 percent less likely to suffer a nonfatal stroke, and nearly 17 percent less likely to die from cardiovascular-related causes. Also see Tip 6.

In a study of 1,200 participants, only 10 percent of those taking aspirin suffered severe strokes, compared with 15 percent of non-users. Those who took just a single aspirin in the week before they suffered an ischemic stroke were significantly less likely to sustain severe stroke-related damage.

IMPORTANT: Check with your doctor before starting any new medications, including aspirin therapy.

Sign up at the World Health Network, www.worldhealth.net, the website of the A4M, for the FREE BioTech e-Newsletter, which shares insights on how you can live longer and better.

38

A Fishy Proposition

"Fatty" fish, rich in essential fatty acids (omega-3 fats), which help to lower cholesterol and prevent blood platelets from sticking to artery walls, have gained much positive attention as health-promoting foods. Some fish should be avoided due to high levels of the potential cancer-causing agent methylmercury. To shop smart for fish, heed the following:

- **Salmon** (both farmed and wild) is especially low in methylmercury. However, compared with the wild version, farmed salmon (due to the feed they receive) may contain as much as sixteen times the level of PCBs, an industrial pollutant linked to cancer, neurological impairment, and developmental delays in children.

- **Flounder, cod, and haddock** are also low in methylmercury. They are also great sources of low-fat protein and are high in the B vitamins.

- **Trout, tuna, and halibut**, while rich in omega-3s, iron, and magnesium, are also fairly high in methylmercury. Limit your consumption.

- **Swordfish and shark** are extremely high in methylmercury. It's best to totally avoid them.

"Govern a great nation as you would cook a small fish. Do not overdo it."

—LAO-TZU, FATHER OF TAOISM

39

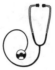

Drink and Thrive

Alcohol in moderation promotes cardiovascular health by boosting concentrations of good cholesterol and inhibiting the formation of dangerous blood clots. Additional compounds in red wine seem to benefit the heart and blood vessels. Drinking alcohol also appears to guard against macular degeneration, an incurable eye disease.

In moderation, alcohol can also help sustain brain function. A Netherlands study tracked 5,395 men and women ages fifty-five and older who were free of dementia (abnormal mental deterioration in old age) at the start of the study. Those categorized as "moderate drinkers" (having one to three alcoholic beverages each day) showed only 58 percent of the risk of dementia calculated for nondrinkers.

Teetotalers may wish to try the nutritional supplement resveratrol, the active therapeutic ingredient in wine.

Sign up at the World Health Network, www.worldhealth.net, the website of the A4M, for the FREE BioTech e-Newsletter, which shares insights on how you can live longer and better.

40

Anti-Aging Aid: NSAIDs

Nonsteroidal anti-inflammatory drugs (NSAIDs) reduce inflammation and are effective against pain and fever (they work by inhibiting prostaglandin synthesis). NSAIDs include aspirin, ibuprofen, naproxen, and ketoprofen.

Presently, there are over a dozen ongoing studies that are evaluating NSAIDs for their role in reducing the inflammatory response that may cause or contribute to cancer.

NSAIDs may be beneficial in preventing or treating Alzheimer's disease (AD):

- They have been shown to prevent the buildup of amyloid-beta 42, a protein linked to the disease.

- A study has shown that men and women taking NSAIDs for two years or longer were 80 percent less likely to develop AD (compared with people who used the drugs for shorter periods or those who did not take them at all). In addition, the longer the participants took the drugs, the greater the decrease in their risk of AD.

IMPORTANT: Check with your doctor before starting any new medications, including NSAIDs therapy.

📖 *The New Anti-Aging Revolution: Stopping the Clock for a Younger, Sexier, Happier You!* by Ronald Klatz and Robert Goldman (Basic Health Publications, 2003) shares insights on preventive tactics that may promote longevity.

41

Orange You Healthy?

Citrus fruits—oranges, lemons, limes, grapefruit, tangerines, and kumquats—support heart health and may help ward off cancer, stroke, diabetes, and other chronic diseases. Eat one a day to enjoy good health.

Citrus fruit is rich in certain vitamins such as:

- Vitamin C (see Tip 28)

- Folic acid: lowers homocysteine, elevated levels of which are associated with coronary heart disease

- Beta carotene: precursor to vitamin A (see Tip 25)

Citrus fruit is also high in fiber (see Tip 42). Fiber plays an an important role in the prevention of colon cancer.

Sign up at the World Health Network, www.worldhealth.net, the website of the A4M, for the FREE BioTech e-Newsletter, which shares insights on how you can live longer and better.

42

Fiber, the Anti-Fat

Fiber soaks up fat. A high-fiber diet can improve your digestion, relieve the strain on your liver and gall bladder, and reduce your risk of large bowel cancer, gallstones, diabetes, arteriosclerosis, colitis, hemorrhoids, hernia, and varicose veins. Your body will benefit from both soluble fiber (sources include dried beans, oats, barley, apples, citrus fruits, and potatoes) and insoluble fiber (found in whole grains, wheat bran, cereals, seeds, and the skins of many fruits and vegetables). Aim for the U.S. Department of Agriculture's recommended intake of 25–30 grams of fiber daily.

The New Anti-Aging Revolution: Stopping the Clock for a Younger, Sexier, Happier You! by Ronald Klatz and Robert Goldman (Basic Health Publications, 2003) shares insights on preventive tactics that may promote longevity.

43

Hormone Health: Human Growth Hormone

Starting at age twenty or so, the body's level of human growth hormone (HGH) begins to decline, so that by the time we are age sixty-five, many of us have little or no HGH. The decline of HGH is accompanied by many of the miseries we associate with aging, from saggy skin to a potbelly, to a lack of vitality.

You can increase your HGH level naturally, through exercise. HGH seems to be released in response to particularly intense and strenuous activity. Weight lifting or resistance exercise, two or three times a week, is particularly effective. Include strenuous lifting (loads you can lift only six times), as well as lower body workouts (such as leg lifts, for at least half your workout time). Of course, check with your doctor before undertaking any strenuous exercise.

Numerous clinical studies have shown that HGH can help men and women gain lean body mass, lose fat mass, and improve markers of heart health. A number of additional studies have found that restoring HGH levels to that of a more youthful state can help people with quality of life, maintain their independence, and reduce the number of visits to the doctor or hospital.

Visit the World Health Network at www.worldhealth.net, the website of the A4M, and use the interactive directory to locate a qualified anti-aging physician and/or clinic in your geographic area.

44

Spice Up for a Long Life

For years, scientists have been tapping our kitchens for creative ways to ward off disease and discomfort. Capsaicin, the main chemical in chili pepper, is used in topical creams to provide relief from arthritis. Allicin, the main ingredient in garlic, can reduce cholesterol and blood pressure when consumed in large quantities.

The latest spice to make it from a kitchen flavor to a health helper is curcumin, which gives the curry spice turmeric its yellow color.

- **Curcumin may help protect against Alzheimer's disease.** This spice triggers production of a protein that fights free-radical damage in the brain.

- **Curcumin may help treat skin cancer.** In a 2005 study by University of Texas Anderson Cancer Center, researchers treated melanoma cell lines with curcumin to cause decreased cell viability and induce cell death in tumor cells.

- **Curcumin halts the spread of breast cancer.** In a 2005 study by scientists also at the University of Texas, curcumin stopped breast cancer from spreading in a mouse model.

Curcumin is also being tested for its therapeutic potential in multiple myeloma and pancreatic cancer, and also for its value in preventing oral cancers. In addition, a university in the United Kingdom received funding in 2005 to study the effects of curcumin on cancers of the gastrointestinal tract.

"Before eating, always take a little time to thank the food."
—AMERICAN INDIAN PROVERB

45

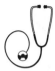

Sunshine for Strength

Roll up your sleeves and enjoy five to fifteen minutes of sunshine each day. The body needs this exposure in order to manufacture vitamin D (skin cells derive it from sunshine). Vitamin D enhances the absorption of calcium from the intestine and the utilization of calcium and phosphorus in the body, so sunshine indirectly contributes to maintaining strong and healthy bones. Keep other body parts covered with sunscreen (SPF 15 or higher) or clothing, and limit the unprotected exposure to fifteen minutes.

The New Anti-Aging Revolution: Stopping the Clock for a Younger, Sexier, Happier You! by Ronald Klatz and Robert Goldman (Basic Health Publications, 2003) shares insights on preventive tactics that may promote longevity.

46

Hormone Health: DHEA

Dehydroepiandrosterone (DHEA) is the most abundant hormone in the human body. It is involved in the manufacture of testosterone, estrogen, progesterone, and corticosterone. The decline of DHEA with age parallels that of HGH (see Tip 43), so by the age of sixty-five, our bodies make only 10 to 20 percent of what they did at age twenty.

DHEA supplementation has been shown in various clinical studies to enhance the immune response against infection. It also has been reported to be valuable against cancer, coronary artery disease, and osteoporosis. DHEA also increases muscle mass and reduces fat mass. DHEA has also been found to increase insulin sensitivity, so it may be valuable in treating diabetes. Because brain tissue contains five to six times more DHEA than any other tissue in the body, some research has found that DHEA supplementation may help protect against Alzheimer's disease.

In addition, DHEA may help stimulate HGH (see Tip 43). Scientists suspect that by restoring the levels of DHEA, the liver may be prompted to produce more IGF-1 (a marker of HGH levels) or to generate more HGH receptors.

Visit the World Health Network at www.worldhealth.net, the website of the A4M, and use the interactive directory to locate a qualified anti-aging physician and/or clinic in your geographic area.

47

Safety Driven

According to the U.S. National Highway Transportation Safety Administration, automobile crashes were the number-one cause of death of Americans ages three through thirty-three. For ages thirty-four through forty-four, car crashes were the third leading cause of death in the United States.

Don't assume that massive vehicles deliver massive protection: there is more to safety than just brute strength during a collision. Instead of automatically buying the largest possible vehicle, look instead at its overall safety profile (see the website below).

Five Star Crash Test and Rollover Ratings are searchable by automobile class, year, make, and model, at www.safercar.gov, a website of the U.S. National Highway Transportation Safety Administration (NHTSA).

48

Hormone Health for Men: Testosterone

Known best as the "sex drive" hormone in men, testosterone levels in men decrease gradually over time, due to factors such as reduced activity, nutritional deficiency, diabetes, and HGH deficiency. This phenomenon is sometimes referred to as andropause. By age sixty, many men have less than half the level of testosterone as they did when they were in their teens.

While testosterone replacement therapy (TRT) can improve erectile function and libido, testosterone is one of the most important anti-aging medications because it has a multitude of additional and noteworthy benefits, including the ability to:

- Increase lean body mass

- Decrease fat mass

- Improve cholesterol profile, including to decrease "bad" cholesterol (LDL)

- Reduce bone fractures

- Improve cognitive functions, including visual spatial perception

- Improve mood, including remission of depression

Visit the World Health Network at www.worldhealth.net, the website of the A4M, and use the interactive directory to locate a qualified anti-aging physician and/or clinic in your geographic area.

49

Savor the Crust

The crusts of bread—and bread-type foods, like pizza—may have cancer-fighting potential. Baking flour changes the amino acid lysine into a compound called pronyl-lysine.

Not only does the pronyl-lysine help darken and sweeten a bread's crust, but it also activates enzymes that inactivate free radicals. Pronyl-lysine is eight times more abundant in cooked crusts than in the uncooked dough.

"Better half a loaf than no bread."
—WILLIAM CAMDEN,
ENGLISH ANTIQUARIAN AND HISTORIAN

50

When Every Drop Counts

Donating your blood can actually do you more good than anyone else who might receive it. Excess iron is thought to be a leading contributor to cancer and heart attacks. An excessive level of iron in your body is one of the most potent ways that your body oxidizes, or prematurely ages. (Think of your body as an apple, and the iron causing the discoloration when the fruit is exposed to air.)

Nearly all adult men carry excess iron, as do many postmenopausal women. These two groups of people may benefit from regularly donating their blood (one to six times per year, depending on their iron overload status). Women who still have periods have lower iron levels, as iron is lost during monthly menstruation.

Sign up at the World Health Network, www.worldhealth.net, the website of the A4M, for the FREE BioTech e-Newsletter, which shares insights on how you can live longer and better.

51

Hormone Health for Women: Estrogen & Progesterone

Replenishing the hormones that decline in menopause may help alleviate some of its symptoms. For these women, either combination hormone replacement therapy (HRT, as estrogen with progesterone) or estrogen replacement therapy (ERT) may be appropriate.

As part of a hormone replacement program for menopause, estrogen has been shown in clinical studies to:

- Replenish bone density

- Reduce coronary artery disease and risk of heart attack

- Reduce the risk of death from stroke

- Reduce the risk of colon cancer

- Improve mood (also may lift depression)

- Promote collagen content in skin, to maintain skin thickness and reduce wrinkles

- Improve carbohydrate metabolism and insulin resistance

- Ease menopause-related memory difficulties and may protect against Alzheimer's disease

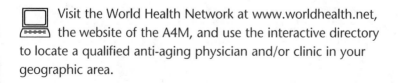 Visit the World Health Network at www.worldhealth.net, the website of the A4M, and use the interactive directory to locate a qualified anti-aging physician and/or clinic in your geographic area.

52

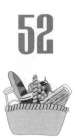

Sweet Heart

In 2005, researchers at Athens Medical School in Greece found that dark chocolate may decrease key markers of cardiovascular performance implicated in heart disease, high blood pressure, and stroke.

In the study, consumption of dark chocolate decreased wave reflections, exerted a beneficial effect on the lining of blood vessels and the lymphatic system, and did not stiffen arteries. Citing the high flavonoid (a type of antioxidant) content in dark chocolate, along with its observed ability to dilate (relax) arteries after consumption, the researchers concluded that "Chocolate may exert a protective effect on the cardiovascular system." Previous research by University of California–Davis scientists found that as little as a handful (25 grams) of semi-sweet chocolate chips caused an increase in blood levels of flavonoids.

"The superiority of chocolate, both for health and nourishment, will soon give it the same preference over tea and coffee in America which it has in Spain . . ."

—THOMAS JEFFERSON, 3RD U.S. PRESIDENT

53

Hormone Health: Melatonin

Melatonin is most notably known as the hormone of sleep: it is produced in the dark by the pineal gland in the brain. Melatonin production peaks when we are age ten or younger, and decreases sharply as we age.

Melatonin supplementation has been shown to:

- Be valuable in resetting the biological clocks of international and transcontinental travelers. As a result, melatonin can combat jet lag and restore restful sleeping patterns in frequent flyers.

- Act as a natural sleeping aid. Compared with prescription sleeping medications, melatonin does not suppress dream (REM-cycle) sleep.

- Lower blood cholesterol in people with elevated cholesterol levels.

- Be a potent scavenger of free radicals, thereby demonstrating value against heart disease, stroke, and cancer.

- Improve sexual drive and performance.

- Increase levels of DHEA (see Tip 46) and IGF-1 (a marker of HGH, see Tip 43).

The New Anti-Aging Revolution: Stopping the Clock for a Younger, Sexier, Happier You! by Ronald Klatz and Robert Goldman (Basic Health Publications, 2003) shares insights on preventive tactics that may promote longevity.

54

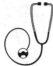

Screenings Save Lives

Age-appropriate screening tests lead the list among all the things you can do to prevent yourself from getting sick. Screening tests can find diseases early when they are easier to treat. The age at which you will start having regularly scheduled screenings will vary, based on your sex, your age, your medical and family history, and other factors.

Men should have the following screenings:

- **Cholesterol check**—At least every five years, starting at age thirty-five. If you smoke or have diabetes, or if heart disease runs in your family, start having your cholesterol checked at age twenty.

- **Blood pressure reading**—At least every two years.

- **Colorectal cancer test**—Starting at age fifty. Your doctor can help you decide which test is right for you. How often you need to be tested will depend on which test you have.

- **Diabetes test**—If you have high blood pressure or high cholesterol.

- **Depression test**—If you've felt "down," sad, or hopeless, and have felt little interest or pleasure in doing things for two weeks straight.

- **Tests for sexually transmitted diseases**—As appropriate.

- **Prostate cancer screening**—Prostate-specific antigen (PSA) test, digital rectal examination (DRE), and/or ultrasound screening. Year to start and frequency are dependent on individual's risk factors for Prostate cancer; consult your physician.

Women should have the following screenings:

- **Cholesterol check**—Starting at age forty-five. If you smoke or have diabetes, or if heart disease runs in your family, start having your cholesterol checked at age twenty.

- **Blood pressure reading**—At least every two years.

- **Breast cancer test**—Mammogram every one to two years beginning at age forty.

- **Cervical cancer test**—Pap smear every one to three years if you have been sexually active or are older than twenty-one (see Tip 18).

- **Colorectal cancer test**—Starting at age fifty. Your doctor can help you decide which test is right for you. How often you need to be tested will depend on which test you have.

- **Diabetes test**—If you have high blood pressure or high cholesterol.

- **Depression test**—If you've felt "down," sad, or hopeless, and have felt little interest or pleasure in doing things for two weeks straight.

- **Osteoporosis test**—Bone density test at age sixty-five to screen for osteoporosis (thinning of the bones). If you are between the ages of sixty and sixty-four and weigh 154 pounds or less, talk to your doctor about whether you should be tested.

- **Chlamydia test and tests for other sexually transmitted diseases**—As appropriate.

Both men and women should have the following screenings:

- **Hearing test**—Annually starting at age fifty, when risk of hearing loss rises.

- **Vision test**—Annually starting at age forty-five, when vision problems often begin.

- **Dental checkup**—Visit your dentist once or twice a year for routine care (see Tip 116).

The New Anti-Aging Revolution: Stopping the Clock for a Younger, Sexier, Happier You! by Ronald Klatz and Robert Goldman (Basic Health Publications, 2003) shares insights on preventive tactics that may promote longevity.

55

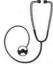

Be Travel Wise, Not Travel Weary

In the United States alone, in 2002, approximately 628 million trips were made by travelers on commercial airplanes. So, it's not too difficult to imagine how easy it could be to become sick while in an airport or aboard an aircraft. To keep the skies friendly to your health, consider following these ten travel-savvy tips:

1. **Wear loose clothing.** If you feel bloated after disembarking from a plane, it's because the low air pressure (8,000 feet, or 2,438 meters, inside the jet cabin) makes our bodies swell up.

2. **Keep your fluids up.** While in flight, drink 8 ounces (236 ml) of water during every hour. Cabin air is notoriously dry (0 to 2% humidity). Be sure to take the flight attendants up on their offers of bottled water during your flight. Avoid tap water on airplanes. It is treated with mild detergents, and no regulatory standards are in effect for commercial aircraft water tanks.

3. **Sip smart.** Avoid alcohol and caffeinated beverages—which act as diuretics. Alcohol's intoxication effect also is more pronounced when consumed in the rarefied atmosphere of air travel.

4. **Skip the airline food.** Snacks are loaded with salt. Airline meals are typically high in fat and preservatives. Brown bag something to tide you over until you reach your destination.

5. **Wiggle a little.** While seated, do some isometric exercises (contract and relax muscles from head to toe). Stand up at your seat to help reduce swelling in the legs and feet. Walk the length of the plane at least once during the flight.

6. **Grab some ZZZs.** To maximize your chances of falling and staying asleep on the flight, you might want to bring a few supplies: earplugs, eye mask, neck pillow, sweater, and cotton socks.

7. **Speak up.** Clammy skin, impaired vision, and difficulty concentrating may be a result of a lack of fresh, oxygenated air being supplied to the cabin. A lack of air results in lack of oxygen to the brain, a medical condition called "hypoxia," which may trigger dizziness, headaches, chest pain, nausea, fatigue, and other unpleasant effects. Newer jets have been designed with less fresh air capacity for passengers; but most of us can attest to having difficulty with the quality or quantity of air on most flights we've endured. Passengers can ask for "air packs" to be turned on and "recirculation fans" to be turned off. It is standard operating procedure for pilots to turn off 30% of the air supply until a passenger complains, since it costs $80 per hour for a 747 to run a single air pack.

8. **Humidify yourself.** At check-in, mist your nasal passages, then put the spray away in your checked luggage.

9. **Grease up.** At check-in, coat the inside of your nostrils with edible oil (corn, olive, jojoba, almond, or similar) to help block the spread of airborne germs (then put the oil away in your checked luggage). Avoid petroleum-based products and synthetic chemicals.

10. **Submerge yourself upon arrival.** After landing, dive into a pool, ocean, lake, hot tub, or bath. Bathing when dehydrated will replenish moisture right through your pores. It will also relax and recharge you so you can enjoy your first outing of the trip.

Infection Protection: How to Fight the Germs That Make You Sick by Ronald Klatz and Robert Goldman (HarperCollins, 2002) shares insights on how to minimize germs in everyday settings.

56

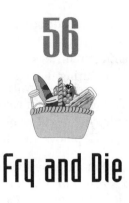

Fry and Die

Avoid eating fried foods for three reasons:

1 All fried foods can contain trans fatty acids (trans fat), formed when vegetable oils are hardened in the cooking process, which hardens arteries. Trans fat increases blood levels of "bad" cholesterol (LDL) and lowers "good" cholesterol (HDL). Trans fats have been shown to contribute to the risk of type 2 diabetes and heart disease.

2 Fried foods often use vegetable oils (nut and seed oils such as canola, soybean, safflower, and corn), which can become rancid and produce large amounts of free radicals that can damage cells, possibly contributing to inflammatory diseases, cancer, obesity, and aging itself.

3 Fried foods contain high levels of a chemical called acrylamide, a byproduct of cooking foods at high temperatures. Acrylamide is a potentially cancer-causing chemical, and also has been shown to be neurotoxic, causing damage to the nervous system in people exposed to the chemical at work. Acrylamide has been found particularly in high-carbohydrate foods cooked at high temperatures.

> *"Our lives are not in the lap of the gods,*
> *but in the lap of our cooks."*
>
> —LIN YUTANG, CHINESE WRITER

57

Burnt Is Bad

Charbroiling meats so they have a dark crust can change proteins and amino acids into substances that can alter the consumer's DNA. Cooking meats at very high temperatures for long periods of time can also be risky.

The Iowa Women's Health Study found that women who consistently ate very well-done meats were 4.6 times more likely to have breast cancer (compared with those who ate meats cooked medium or rare). Adding rosemary extract to precooked ground beef may cut carcinogens (cancer-causing compounds) from forming during grilling by up to 80 percent, reports Kansas Sate University researchers in 2005.

The New Anti-Aging Revolution: Stopping the Clock for a Younger, Sexier, Happier You! by Ronald Klatz and Robert Goldman (Basic Health Publications, 2003) shares insights on preventive tactics that may promote longevity.

58

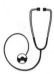

Ring, Ring . . . Radiation Calling

Worldwide cellular connections exceed 2 billion. One in three people around the globe are wired up via mobile connections. With such broad usage, cellular phone technology is giving rise to important questions about possible long-term health consequences associated with its use. Cellular phones emit low frequency electromagnetic fields (EMFs), which have been linked to health conditions such as:

- General malaise

- Immune-system dysfunction

- Male sexual and reproductive issues

- Changes in the central nervous system and cardiovascular system

- Changes in memory, cognition, attention, and other brain functions

- Elevations in blood pressure

- Skin damage

- Changes in red blood cells

Because of the immense numbers of present and projected users, some scientists and public health experts are worried that even if only a small percentage are adversely affected, that could still equate to a public health issue of epidemic proportions. We offer these tips to minimize your cellular phone radiation exposure:

1. Call Length and Frequency

A number of the scientific studies have shown a correlation between the length of calls and/or frequency of use with biological changes.

 TIP Reserve cellular phone use for short, necessary conversations. Keep incoming mobile phone calls as brief as possible and return your calls on a corded phone.

2. Distance

The concentration of radiation emissions is directly related to the power of the emitting device. The farther you can put yourself from the cellular phone handset, the less emissions you will receive. Radiation from all sources obeys the inverse square law. That is, the further you are from the source, the less intense your exposure to the radiation. In fact, it drops off with the square of your distance from the source.

 TIP Many cellular phones now have a "speakerphone" option, permitting a substantial distancing between the user and the handset during conversations.

3. Phone Antenna

The type of antenna that is on your cellular phone may contribute to the amount of radiation it emits. Stubby antennae cannot be extended and have been shown to be worse than extendable antenna because they concentrate energy into the user's brain.

 TIP Select a phone with an extendable antenna.

4. Signal Path

The steel construction of vehicles and buildings creates an electrical shielding effect ("Faraday cage"). As a result, using a cellular phone inside an enclosed vehicle or building causes the phone to increase the power output it needs to establish a connection, receive signals, and transmit signals, all of which cause increased radiation emissions. A presentation by the United Kingdom's House of Commons Science and Technology System reported that using a cellular phone inside an enclosed vehicle can cause radiation levels to rise by ten times.

 TIP If using the cellular phone inside a vehicle, open the window or door (if not in motion). This will improve the path for the cellular phone signals and possibly reduce the phone's need to increase its power level.

5. Phone Mode

The highest cellular phone emissions occur when the phone is establishing a connection with a base station. When using the phone in a mobile setting, the phone is constantly reestablishing its base station connection. The emissions in the mobile setting are further compounded by signal path issues (see preceding tip).

 TIP When inside a vehicle, avoid keeping the cellular phone handset turned on unless you are expecting an incoming call or making a call.

6. Carrying the Phone

Avoid keeping the cellular phone (when switched on) adjacent to your body. In particular, do not keep it in on-mode in clothing pockets or clipped to the waist. The soft tissues of the body—namely heart, liver, kidneys, intestines, and reproductive organs—are very vulnerable to penetration by radiation, more so than the brain (which is protected to a degree by the skull). According to a report to the Economic Union, three sudden deaths occurred from colon cancer among members of a secret surveillance unit of the former United Kingdom's Royal Ulster Constabulary, all of whom had worn radio or microwave transmitters in the lower part of their backs for extended periods of time.

TIP Women: carry your phone in a purse that is carried away from the body. Men: do not carry the phone in the on-mode in your chest, jacket, or pants pockets.

7. Eyeglass Wearers

The House of Commons Science and Technology System report also found that cellular phone users who wear metal-rimmed glasses intensify their exposure to radiation emissions to the eye by 20 percent and to the head by 6.3 percent.

 TIP Take glasses off when making or receiving cellular phone calls, or wear contact lenses when using the cell phone.

8. Proximity to Base Stations

The number of "cells" (zones of service) in the geographic area, in addition to the proximity of the cellular phone to a base station, factor into the power necessary for the phone to establish a connection and receive and transmit signals. The fewer the number of cells, and the farther apart the base stations, the greater the power (and radiation emission) necessary to maintain contact with the network.

TIP Many cellular phones can display the signal level at which they are operating when turned on. When receiving or making a call, take note of the reported signal level. If it is weak, keep the call short and continue it later on a corded phone or when you reach an area where the signal level is stronger.

The New Anti-Aging Revolution: Stopping the Clock for a Younger, Sexier, Happier You! by Ronald Klatz and Robert Goldman (Basic Health Publications, 2003) shares insights on preventive tactics that may promote longevity.

59

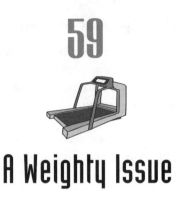

A Weighty Issue

Obesity and overweight are determined by the body mass index (BMI)—a measure of body fat based on height and weight. You can calculate your BMI by using the interactive U.S. National Heart, Lung, and Blood Institute's Body Mass Index calculator at www. nhlbi.nih.gov/health. Look under "Health Assessment Tools," and select "Body Mass Index (BMI) Calculator." It has options for both standard and Metric measures. A BMI over 25 is defined as overweight, and a BMI of over 30 as obese.

Overweight and obesity can be life threatening, in that excess weight can result in:

- Cardiovascular disease

- Type 2 diabetes

- Cancer of the breast, colon, prostate, endometrium, kidney, and gallbladder

Overweight or obesity can also significantly hamper quality of life. Excess weight is associated with respiratory difficulties, chronic musculoskeletal problems, skin problems, and infertility. Chronic overweight and obesity contribute significantly to osteoarthritis, a major cause of disability in adults.

"Globally, there are more than 1 billion overweight adults, at least 300 million of them obese."
—WORLD HEALTH ORGANIZATION

60

Berry Smart

Berries, in general, show great promise in slowing and reversing many of the degenerative diseases associated with an aging brain. With a high ORAC (oxygen radical absorbance capacity) value, blueberries, blackberries, strawberries, and raspberries can offset the free-radical damage that can cause vascular damage, which in turn can lead to memory and thinking impairments.

In particular, blueberries are emerging as one of the best foods that protect brain health. Scientists from the Universidad Nacional Autonoma de Mexico have found that rats fed a blueberry-enriched diet had lower levels of NF-kappaB, a protein involved in brain aging. High levels of NF-kappaB are associated with poor memory.

Another animal study showed that consumption of blueberries reduced brain cell loss and improved recovery of movement following a stroke. In a study by researchers at the U.S. National Institute on Aging, blueberries were found to help lessen some of the functional damage caused by brain injury. In the future, consumption of blueberries and other berries may represent a significant positive advancement that can help with brain aging, Alzheimer's disease, and other neurological disorders.

*"We must always have old memories
and young hopes."*
—Arsène Houssaye, French novelist

61

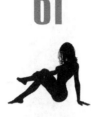

Sin of the Skin #1:
Fine Lines and Wrinkles

Humans express feelings, and as such, these emotions become the fine lines seen with aging. Squinting leads to crow's feet (lines radiating from the corners of the eyes), frowning causes frown lines (furrows between the eyebrows), and laughing leads to laugh lines (arc-shapes around the mouth). Wrinkles are a result of age-related weakening of the skin's collagen and elastin, the fibers that keep the skin firm in youth.

To prevent and minimize fine lines and wrinkles, wear sunblock with an SPF 15 or greater whenever you venture out of doors for more than fifteen minutes. Skin moisturizers containing pregnenolone, a hormone, may help to hydrate the skin and improve visible wrinkles.

In 2005, Canadian researchers proved that beta glucan, the soluble fiber found in the cell walls of oat kernels and an ingredient in some skincare products, can penetrate the skin and reduce the appearance of wrinkles.

> *"If wrinkles must be written upon our brows,*
> *let them not be written upon the heart.*
> *The spirit should not grow old."*
> —JAMES GARFIELD, 20TH U.S. PRESIDENT

62

Cure a Lagging Libido

Libido, or sexual desire and arousal, is a symphony of biochemical signals:

- **DHEA**—In animals, DHEA promotes libido, orgasms, and sex appeal (see Tip 46).

- **Dopamine**—A neurotransmitter, it is a primary brain chemical responsible for desire and arousal. By prompting the release of luteinizing hormone-releasing hormone (LHRH), dopamine causes men to produce testosterone.

- **Testosterone**—The key hormone necessary for sexual desire in both men and women, and is critical for men to achieve erection.

- **Oxytocin**—A protein produced in the brain, it reaches peak levels during orgasm.

After ruling out other possible causes of decreased sexual desire, a qualified physician can identify whether biochemical imbalances play a contributing role.

Visit the World Health Network at www.worldhealth.net, the website of the A4M, and use the interactive directory to locate an anti-aging physician with experience in treating sexual dysfunction in your geographic area.

63

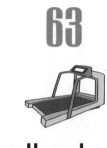

Use It or Lose It

Substantial health benefits occur with regular physical activity that is aerobic in nature (such as thirty to sixty minutes of brisk walking, five or more days of the week). Additional health benefits can be gained through greater amounts of physical activity, but even small amounts of activity are healthier than a sedentary lifestyle. Regular exercise in middle age can help men and women prolong their physical prowess as they grow older.

A 2005 study by University College London found that among 6,400 adults between the ages of thirty-nine and sixty-three, those who could be categorized as "sufficiently active" at the start of the study were more likely to be free of physical limitations nine years later. "Sufficiently active" study subjects were those men and women who engaged in two and a half hours of moderate exercise (such as biking and leisurely swimming) or one hour of vigorous activity (swimming laps and running, for example) each week.

After nine years of regular aerobic physical activity, sufficiently active adults were less likely to have physical problems that kept them from playing sports, lifting heavy objects, or being able to perform routine activities such as climbing stairs or bathing. The researchers conclude that "This study shows that regular physical activity appears to be critical to preserving high physical function in relatively fit, healthy, middle-aged men and women."

*"More than 60 percent of the global population
is not sufficiently active."*

—WORLD HEALTH ORGANIZATION

64

A Healthy Curiosity

In 2005, researchers from the University of Alberta in Canada found that for 90 percent of the population, keeping the brain sharp as we age can be as simple as being and staying mentally inquisitive. The team found that people who are curious at a young age are more likely to be mentally active, and stay that way, as they age. In addition, people in their seventies and eighties who started incorporating activities to improve mental capacity at those ages could enjoy similar benefits to brain health.

Some of the best activities that keep the mind active and curious include reading, traveling, memorizing poetry, playing card games, doing crossword puzzles, learning how to play a musical instrument, taking classes, and surfing the Internet.

> *"The mind is its own place, and in itself can make
> a heaven of hell, a hell of heaven."*
>
> —JOHN MILTON, ENGLISH POET

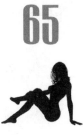

65

Sin of the Skin #2: Age Spots

Blotches in which small patches of skin appear to have a different color than the main skin area become common as we age. It is important for you and your dermatologist to watch your skin discolorations carefully. For warts and liver spots (also known as age spots), which are harmless, try cosmetics and skincare products containing one or more of these ingredients:

- **Hydroquinone**, an antioxidant that has been found to be helpful in breaking down and preventing the accumulation of browned pigment cells that form age spots (lipofuscin).

- **Kojic acid**, which is derived from mushrooms and soy, and has been used by the Japanese to fight age spots.

- *Glycyrrhiza glabra*, an herb that breaks up clumps of brown skin cells so that they can be shed by the body's natural cycle of exfoliation, and by fighting free radicals, which contribute to the production of lipofuscin.

IMPORTANT: Some skin discolorations can be harmful. A small flat brown spot can become cancerous, especially if its shape changes or if it starts to itch, which may be early signs of melanoma, a deadly form of skin cancer. See your doctor if you experience these symptoms. The U.S. National Cancer Institute addresses melanoma at its "What You Need to Know About Melanoma" webpage, www.cancer.gov/cancerinfo/wyntk/melanoma, where you can learn about the signs and symptoms.

Visit the World Health Network at www.worldhealth.net, the website of the A4M, and use the interactive directory to locate a qualified anti-aging physician and/or clinic in your geographic area.

66

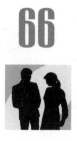

Love Together, Live Longer

Researchers from Victoria University in Australia tracked 3,000 eld-erly men and women for fifteen years, and reported in 2005 that married men lived, on average, eleven months longer than their single counterparts. Marriage, however, was found to have little effect on the life span of married women. A previous study, by a team at University of Victoria in Canada, that followed 9,775 men and women, found that men and women report a decrease in phys-ical or mental health when they ended a marriage or stopped liv-ing with their partner.

Some scientists have put forth a theory called the "marriage pro-tection hypothesis," suggesting that married couples improve their health by providing each other with social and financial support, and by monitoring each other's health behaviors.

"If thou wouldst marry wisely,
marry thine equal."
—OVID, ROMAN POET

67

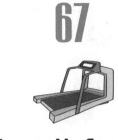

Strength for Life

While aerobic exercise (see Tip 63) is important to keep weight within a healthy range and improve the cardiovascular system, strength training is just as important. Strength training, which is also referred to as resistance training, enables men and women at any age to improve their overall health and fitness by increasing muscular strength, endurance, and bone density. This particular type of physical activity also improves insulin sensitivity and glucose metabolism.

Studies show that even men and women in their nineties who took up weight training increased muscle mass and strengthened bones, key improvements in preventing falls and injuries and encouraging continued independent living. Yet, only 11 percent of older adults meet strength training recommendations. The vast majority of older adults are missing opportunities to improve their health through strength training. At a minimum, try for twenty minutes of aerobic exercise (see Tip 63) along with ten minutes of weight training, four times a week. Be sure to check with your doctor before beginning any new exercise program.

> *"Champions aren't made in gyms. Champions are made from something they have deep inside them: A desire, a dream, a vision. The will must be stronger than the skill."*
>
> —MUHAMMAD ALI, AMERICAN BOXER

68

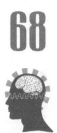

Give Back to Get Healthy

Giving your time to help others can pay off in real health benefits for you. Volunteering increases your cognitive and mental well-being, promoting skills such as thinking, reasoning, remembering, imagining, and learning words. Volunteering helps keep the brain engaged, which helps protect the memory as you age. Volunteers are also physically healthy.

Several studies show that people who volunteer have fewer medical problems and stay physically active, thereby possibly reducing their risk of heart disease, diabetes, and other cardiovascular problems.

> *"There is no exercise better for the heart*
> *than reaching down and lifting people up."*
> —JOHN ANDREW HOLMES, JR.,
> AMERICAN PHYSICIAN AND WRITER

69

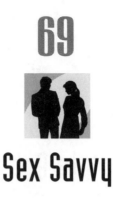

Sex Savvy

We've all heard the adage that "When you sleep with someone, you sleep with everyone they've ever slept with." With regard to the risk of catching an infectious disease from your sex partner, we can only practice—and encourage our partner to practice—safer sex:

- The safest sex is with a disease-free partner in a mutually monogamous relationship.

- Choose your partner carefully. Avoid high-risk groups such as intravenous drug users, men who have sex with other men, and people of either gender with a history of incarceration or who are sexually involved with inmates.

- Know your partner's sex history. You are at risk if your partner has had sex with anyone else in the past three to five years.

- Check your sex partner for warning signs of STDs. A white-coated tongue could signal candidiasis, while a yellowish tinge to the whites of the eyes could indicate hepatitis. Look for open sores or vaginal warts in women, genital warts in men, and anal warts in both sexes. Feel whether lymph nodes (neck and armpit nodes are easiest to find) seem swollen. The lower right side of the abdominal area, where the bulk of the liver is located, as well as the area just below the bottom of the rib cage where the spleen is found, should not be tender to the touch.

> *"Of the delights of this world, man cares most for sexual intercourse. He will go to any length for it— risk fortune, character, reputation, life itself."*
>
> —MARK TWAIN, AMERICAN WRITER

70

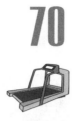

Chores, the Hidden Fatbuster

For men and women of average weight (about 155 pounds, or 70.5 kilograms), everyday chores and tasks can burn off the excess pounds. If you weigh more or less, the caloric expenditures will differ.

- **Taking care of the kids** (dressing or feeding them): 211–246 calories per hour

- **Playing with the kids:** 281–352 calories per hour

- **House cleaning:** 176–317 calories per hour

- **Gardening:** 352 calories per hour

- **Mowing the lawn:** 176–387 calories per hour

- **Moving furniture:** 422 calories per hour

- **Painting or wallpapering the house:** 317 calories per hour

- **Shoveling snow (by hand):** 422 calories per hour

- **Sweeping the driveway:** 281 calories per hour

> *"Health lies in labor, and there is no royal road to it but through toil."*
>
> —WENDELL PHILLIPS,
> AMERICAN ABOLITIONIST

71

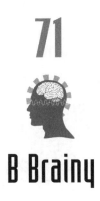

B Brainy

Homocysteine, a marker for cardiovascular disease risk, is associated with lower scores on tests that evaluate cognitive skills—thinking, reasoning, remembering, imagining, and learning words.

In a 2005 analysis of data from the Veterans Affairs Normative Aging Study, tracking men between ages fifty and eighty-five years, researchers at Tufts University found that men with higher blood levels of folate (folic acid), pyridoxine (vitamin B_6), and cobalamin (vitamin B_{12}) were able to retain their verbal skills and spatial perception skills.

High homocysteine levels were found to decrease recall memory skills. To help prevent against age-related mental decline and reduce homocysteine levels, eat leafy green vegetables (rich in folate and B vitamins), and take a vitamin B complex supplement.

"The power of Thought,
the magic of the Mind!"

—LORD BYRON, ANGLO-SCOTTISH POET

72

Sin of the Skin #3: Thin Skin

As we age, the skin becomes papery thin, and suffers from a decrease in oil-gland activity (which also may cause skin to become dry). Largely a function of hormonal decline, you may benefit from a hormone replacement regimen. Consult an anti-aging physician, who will follow these guiding principles to design your hormone replacement therapy (HRT) regimen:

- Use natural, not synthetic, agents.

- Select bioidentical hormones, which the body is able to use safely and efficiently.

- Prescribe proper dosing (as stipulated by laboratory testing for deficits), not supraphysiologic dosing (extremely high doses that often are unjustified by lab testing).

- Conduct regular follow-up office visits and lab tests, to monitor progress.

Visit the World Health Network at www.worldhealth.net, the website of the A4M, and use the interactive directory to locate a qualified anti-aging physician and/or clinic in your geographic area.

73

Kiss of Death

Kissing is a human expression of emotion that can range in intensity from energetic to erotic, platonic to passionate. As sensually enjoyable as the activity may be, kissing exchanges saliva, microbes, and all, from kisser to kissee. Kissing can spread:

- The common cold

- Influenza

- Mononucleosis

- The herpes virus (1 and 2)

- Syphilis

Kissing can also transmit the pathogens that some scientists link to heart disease, stroke, and pneumonia (see Tip 116). Saliva spreads germs, so it is best to avoid kissing with people who have any of the conditions mentioned above.

> *"I wonder what fool it was*
> *that first invented kissing."*
> —JONATHAN SWIFT, ANGLO-IRISH WRITER

74

Age Ain't an Excuse

A study conducted by researchers at the University of Michigan should inspire men and women in their fifties and sixties to become physically active—especially those who have conditions or habits that endanger the heart, like diabetes, high blood pressure, or a smoking habit. Tracking 9,611 older adults, the researchers found that those who were regularly active in their fifties and sixties were 35 percent less likely to die in the next eight years than those who were sedentary. The reduction in the risk of early death was achieved in study participants who engaged in very moderate physical activity (leisurely walking, gardening, and dancing). Even those who were obese had a lower risk of dying if they were regularly active.

The team concluded that "across all ranges of cardiovascular risk, everybody got a benefit from regular activity, but the biggest absolute benefit, the biggest reduction in deaths, was among high risk people." Commenting on their findings, the lead researcher suggested that, in men and women with cardiovascular issues, the risk of remaining sedentary is far greater than the risk of having an acute problem brought on by exercise.

Find a personal trainer specializing in anti-aging sports medicine by contacting the American College of Anti-Aging Sportsmedicine Professionals (ACASP). Call 773-528-4333 or e-mail sports@worldhealth.net.

75

Broccoli on the Brain

Broccoli is high in lignans, a phytoestrogen compound that has been shown to benefit cognitive skills (thinking, reasoning, remembering, imagining, and learning words). A 2005 study by researchers at King's College London revealed that broccoli is also high in glucosinolates, a group of compounds that can halt the decline of the neurotransmitter, acetylcholine, which is necessary for the central nervous system to perform properly (low levels of acetylcholine are common in those with Alzheimer's disease).

If you're not fond of broccoli, try other glucosinolate-rich foods such as potatoes, oranges, apples, radishes, and other cabbage-family vegetables like Brussels sprouts.

"The mind grows by what it feeds on."

—J. G. HOLLAND, AMERICAN NOVELIST AND POET

76

Sin of the Skin #4: Dry Skin

As we age, skin becomes drier. Actually, "xerosis," the medical name for dry skin, affects only the very outermost layer of the epidermis—the stratum corneum. Dry skin causes the skin to become flaky, itchy, or "tight," and discomfort is often the prevailing complaint. Genetics, disease, lifestyle, and the environment can all cause the skin to become dry. Drink one 8-ounce (236-ml) glass of distilled water, with a pinch of sea salt (for electrolytes), every one to two hours that you are awake. By flushing toxins from the body with liquid that is free of deleterious metals and bacteria, you permit your skin to remain well hydrated.

IMPORTANT: Seek medical advice if no obvious cause of dry skin can be identified, as the situation may be caused by an underlying medical problem. Dry skin may arise as a direct result of another dermatological problem, for example dermatitis, eczema, or psoriasis; however, it can also be a sign of hypothyroidism (an underactive thyroid gland). Diabetics should always consult their doctor if they develop signs and symptoms of dry skin (or any other skin complaint), as diabetes can cause serious skin conditions.

Visit the World Health Network at www.worldhealth.net, the website of the A4M, and use the interactive directory to locate a qualified anti-aging physician and/or clinic in your geographic area.

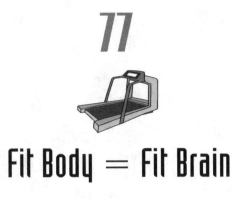

Fit Body = Fit Brain

Physically active adults have higher concentration skills, which may help maintain memory and combat dementia. A study by researchers at Northwestern University Feinberg School of Medicine found that sedentary lifestyles directly contribute to the decline in cognitive abilities and quality of sleep as we age.

In this study, men and women ages sixty-seven to eighty-six, who were functionally independent, participated in a two-week study involving a regimen of thirty minutes of mild physical activity, thirty minutes of social interaction, and a final thirty minutes of mild to moderate physical activity. Sessions began with warm-up stretching and mild to moderate physical activity (walking or stationary upper- and lower-body exercises). The final period of mild to moderate physical activity included rapid walking, calisthenics, or dancing. A ten-minute cool-down concluded the ninety-minute regimen.

At the end of the two-week period, all of the participants demonstrated a 4 to 6 percent improvement in cognitive performance, and improved sleep quality (including deeper sleep and fewer awakenings).

> *"To keep the body in good health is a duty . . .*
> *otherwise we shall not be able to keep*
> *our mind strong and clear."*
>
> —BUDDHA

78

Sin of the Skin #5: Rough Skin

Rough skin is commonly caused by the accumulation of dead skin cells on the skin's surface. These dead cells are usually discarded by the body via a natural process called exfoliation, where newer cells push older skin cells to the surface and the uppermost layer of dead cells flake off to reveal the newer cells underneath. However, for some reason exfoliation does not always happen. The resulting buildup of dead skin cells causes the skin surface to appear bumpy and rough in texture.

Invest in a body brush or a loofah. Body brushing is a good way to stimulate blood circulation, which in turn can help to eliminate toxins, and get rid of dead skin cells. Brush the skin in a circular motion, paying particular attention to the elbows, knees, shoulders, back, and thighs. For the best results, brush every day before bathing or showering.

> *"To the artist there is
> never anything ugly in nature."*
> —AUGUSTE RODIN, FRENCH SCULPTOR

79

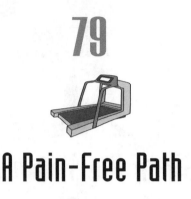

A Pain-Free Path

A 2005 study by researchers at Stanford University tracked 900 adults ages fifty and over for fourteen years. They found that the men and women who routinely exercised were less likely to develop pains in their joints and muscles, as well as rheumatoid arthritis. Men and women who ran, swam, walked briskly, biked, or did aerobics experienced 25 percent less joint and muscle pain. The pain-free men and women who engaged in brisk aerobic exercise completed upwards of six hours of activity a week.

"There are 1,440 minutes in each day,
and 30 of them should be devoted to physical activity."
—U.S. CENTERS FOR DISEASE CONTROL AND PREVENTION

80

Hugs & Snugs

Therapeutic touch is a healing modality employed by health practitioners and nurses to help relieve pain, depression, and anxiety. Various scientific experiments have shown that touch causes measurable and positive physiological changes in both the person doing the touching and the one receiving the touch. Hugging can be considered a two-way version of therapeutic touch. It is a safe alternative to kissing (see Tip 73) and a wholesome, feel-good activity.

Infection Protection: How to Fight the Germs That Make You Sick by Ronald Klatz and Robert Goldman (HarperCollins, 2002) shares insights on how to maintain your sexual health and how to reduce sexually related risks to longevity.

81

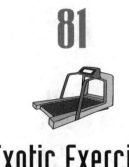

Exotic Exercise

Men and women who are humdrum about exercise might benefit by experimenting with Asian fitness programs.

People ages forty to sixty who practiced Soo Bahk Do, an ancient Korean martial art similar to karate, were found by a group of researchers at the Institute of Technology to be in much better shape after three years (compared with sedentary men and women). Those participating in martial arts enjoyed greater aerobic capacity, muscle strength, and endurance; less body fat; better balance; and increased heart and breathing capacities. Soo Bahk Do also promotes flexibility, strength, speed, and mental focus.

Tai chi, a Chinese exercise dating back to the twelfth century, teaches balance and proper breathing, both of which may become problematic as we age. A study by Emory University School of Medicine found that older people who took part in a fifteen-week tai chi program reduced their risk of falling by more than 47 percent. Many people also report an improved confidence in walking. Tai chi has also been shown to lower blood pressure and improve sleep.

"Your body is precious.
It is our vehicle for awakening.
Treat it with care."
—BUDDHA

82

Sin of the Skin #6: Dull Skin

Up to the age of fourteen, the skin on the face exfoliates naturally every fourteen days. This quick rate of renewal leaves the youngster with a healthy-looking glowing complexion. However, as we get older the rate of natural exfoliation slows down. By the age of twenty-five and over, the skin will exfoliate every twenty-eight days or so. The resulting buildup of dead skin cells can leave the skin looking dull.

Establish a twice-daily skin routine of cleansing, toning, and moisturizing. Look for products that contain alpha and beta hydroxy acids (AHAs and BHAs), because they can help promote the natural process of exfoliation. Those with sensitive skin may wish to opt for products containing poly hydroxy acid (PHA), as it is non-irritating.

*"You can only perceive real beauty
in a person as they get older."*
—ANOUK AIMÉE, FRENCH FILM ACTRESS

83

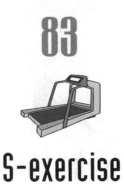

S-exercise

Researchers from the Harvard School of Public Health studied data from the Health Professionals Follow-Up Study, involving 31,742 men ages fifty-three to ninety. They found that men who were physically active reported experiencing better erections. In addition, men who walked briskly for thirty minutes most days of the week reduced their risk of erectile dysfunction by 15 to 20 percent. The researchers posit that exercise, which benefits overall vascular health, has specific value for the small arteries involved in erections, suggesting that "what happens to the penis may be an early warning of what could happen to the heart, such as a heart attack."

An estimated 152 million men worldwide
suffer from erectile dysfunction (ED).
The most common cause of ED is vascular,
accounting for 40 percent of cases.

84

Sex Smarts

Scientists from the Medical Research Center in Germany have suggested that having sex regularly can make people smarter. During foreplay and intercourse, large quantities of adrenaline and hydrocortisone are secreted. These compounds stimulate the gray matter of the brain, which in turn stimulates intellectual activity, the team explains.

"France is now officially the sexiest country with the French having sex 137 times a year, well above the global average of 103. The Japanese have sex the least, averaging 46 times a year."
—GLOBAL SEX SURVEY 2004 BY DUREX CORP.

85

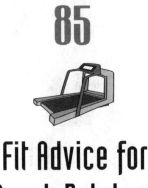

Fit Advice for Couch Potatoes

Men and women who have been inactive for a while should start a physical fitness routine sensibly. Speak with your doctor before embarking on an exercise regimen. Here are some suggestions for the inactive:

- Begin by choosing moderate-intensity activities you enjoy the most. By choosing activities you enjoy, you'll be more likely to stick with them.

- Gradually build up the time spent doing the activity by adding a few minutes every few days or so until you can comfortably perform a minimum recommended amount of activity (thirty minutes per day).

- As the minimum amount becomes easier, gradually increase either the length of time performing an activity or increase the intensity of the activity, or both.

- Vary your activities, both for interest and to broaden the range of benefits.

- Explore new physical activities.

- Reward and acknowledge your efforts.

"To climb steep hills requires slow pace at first."
—WILLIAM SHAKESPEARE, ENGLISH POET AND PLAYWRIGHT

86

Sin of the Skin #7: Acne

Acne, America's number-one skin disease, is caused by a disorder of the sebaceous glands (oil-producing glands in the skin) that blocks pores, thus producing an outbreak of skin lesions we've nicknamed zits, pimples, and other less-flattering names.

Use oil-free skincare products and wear oil-free cosmetics and oil-free sunblock to reduce the risk of clogged pores. Do not pick or squeeze acne eruptions, as doing so may cause the blockage to be pushed further into the skin. If you suffer from acne, use a lotion or gel that contains 2.5 percent benzoyl peroxide to kill off acne-causing bacteria. If you see no improvement in two months, see a dermatologist.

Visit the World Health Network at www.worldhealth.net, the website of the A4M, and use the interactive directory to locate a qualified anti-aging physician and/or clinic in your geographic area.

87

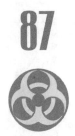

Breakfast as the Best Defense

People who eat breakfast are less likely to catch a cold or the flu, found researchers from Cardiff University in the United Kingdom. The team speculates that a hearty breakfast fuels the immune system with cellular energy. Additionally, people who routinely miss breakfast are more likely to have more stressful, hectic lives, which may weaken immune defenses and increase the chances of getting an infection. Start your day with fresh fruit (oranges or berries) or unsweetened juice, dairy foods (low-fat milk or yogurt), and whole grains (whole-grain hot or cold cereals, whole-wheat toast).

Infection Protection: How to Fight the Germs That Make You Sick by Ronald Klatz and Robert Goldman (HarperCollins, 2002) shares insights on how to maintain your immune system in peak performance, thereby reducing your risks of getting sick due to the pathogens that lurk everywhere.

88

Exercise for a
Great Night's Sleep

Physical exercise promotes faster time to sleep and improves progress through the stages of sleep:

- Moderate aerobic exercise three days a week has been found to promote sound sleep.

- Strength training exercise (including weightlifting) prompts the release of human growth hormone (HGH), rising levels of which at night coincide with sleep (see Tip 43).

- Exercise strengthens bones and joints, thereby helping to alleviate pain that can be bothersome while trying to fall or stay asleep.

NOTE: It is best to avoid exercise for two to four hours before bedtime because of its hormone-releasing—and thus possibly stimulating—effect.

"After the age of 65, 13% of men and 36% of women reported taking more than 30 minutes to fall asleep."
—NATIONAL SLEEP FOUNDATION

89

Don't Pull the Trigger

Stress is an insidious trigger of disease. People who are unable to relieve daily stress suffer a variety of health consequences, most commonly fatigue, frequent headaches, and stomach upset. The emotional response of stress is a function of the release of the hormone cortisol. In times of stress, the adrenal glands atop the kidneys release cortisol. Unfortunately, long-term cortisol release accelerates the aging process. Unrestrained cortisol secretion can inhibit immunity, slow protein synthesis (necessary for tissue repair), lead to loss of nerve cells, brain damage, bone loss, muscle wasting, increased abdominal fat, psychosis, and premature aging and death. Long-term oversecretion of cortisol due to chronic prolonged stress can lead to hypertension and hypoglycemia, both with deadly consequences.

Don't give in to the triggers that start the stress reaction:

- Prepare a list of your daily activities and rank them in order of priority. Accomplish what you can, but don't fret if it all doesn't get done.

- Participate in—and enjoy—the experience of leisure activities. This will reduce the taxing load of stress on the adrenals.

- If you find yourself embroiled with conflicts at work, home, or anywhere else, take the time to resolve the matter.

"Do not take life too seriously.
You will never get out of it alive."

—ELBERT GREEN HUBBARD,
AMERICAN PHILOSOPHER AND WRITER

90

Exercise Away Sickness

People who maintain a physically active lifestyle enjoy the benefits of a stronger immune system into older age. University of Colorado–Boulder researchers found that there is an age-related decline in the antibody responses to signals that elicit the immune response. Physical activity helps to maintain a more optimal T cell–mediated response, and is especially important in those in their fifties, sixties, and beyond, because older people tend to be immunocompromised.

Find a personal trainer specializing in anti-aging sports medicine by contacting the American College of Anti-Aging Sportsmedicine Professionals (ACASP). Call 773-528-4333 or e-mail sports@worldhealth.net.

91

Lower the Lead

A lifetime of low-level exposure to lead in the environment may contribute to mental decline as we age, reported researchers at Harvard School of Public Health in 2005. Tracking 466 men averaging sixty-seven years of age, the team found that the higher the men's level of lead present in the kneecap, a bone marker of cumulative lead exposure, the worse they scored in tests of memory, attention, language, and other mental functions. A separate study by researchers at Brigham and Women's Hospital found that accumulated lead exposure increases the risk of cataracts, a leading cause of age-related blindness. The team tracked 642 men ages sixty and older for five years, finding that those who developed cataracts had increased levels of lead in their bones.

Older people, who are prone to osteoporosis, are particularly vulnerable to the damaging effects of lead because the toxin lodges in bone pores and can be released over a long period of time into the bloodstream, allowing it to damage body tissue.

Lead is no longer present in gasoline and paints available in the United States, but leaded products may be available in other nations, putting those residents at risk. Drinking water may also be a possible source of lead, as the toxin can be introduced via older plumbing.

The New Anti-Aging Revolution: Stopping the Clock for a Younger, Sexier, Happier You! by Ronald Klatz and Robert Goldman (Basic Health Publications, 2003) shares insights on preventive tactics that may promote longevity.

92

Snack and Sleep

Eat for sleep: For dinner or a light nighttime snack, choose foods containing the amino acid tryptophan, from which the body makes serotonin and melatonin, key biochemicals that trigger sleep. Dairy products, beans, poultry, and leafy green vegetables are good sources of tryptophan.

"Many older adults often get less sleep then they need.
One reason is that they often have more trouble
falling asleep. A study of adults over 65 found that
13 percent of men and 36 percent of women
take more than 30 minutes to fall asleep."
—U.S. NIH Department of Senior Health

93

Simple Tips to Manage Stress

Among the ways to reduce your stress levels, some of the top involve being good to yourself. Try to:

- **Avoid negativity:** Poor morale and outlook can be contagious. Avoid people who speak and behave negatively. Rather, stick with friends who find that silver lining and share your enthusiasm for life.

- **Reward yourself with meditation and self-reflection:** Set aside a focused period of quiet time each day during which you contemplate inner peace and mind/body well-being.

- **Enjoy the pleasures of deep breathing:** Clear both mind and body of stress-inducing blockages by fully inhaling and exhaling slowly for ten minutes at a time, three times daily.

"Make up your mind to be happy.
Learn to find pleasure in the simple things."
—ROBERT LOUIS STEVENSON, SCOTTISH NOVELIST

94

Breathe Easy

People spend about 90 percent of their time indoors. Consequently, the risks to health may be greater due to exposure to air pollution indoors than outdoors. Cut down on indoor triggers of allergies and asthma by following these simple tips:

- Remove pets from the home and thoroughly clean to eliminate their dander.

- Opt for leather furniture rather than upholstered pieces, since leather is an impervious material that is resistant to breeding dust mites.

- Eliminate carpet and drapes.

- Dust both vertical and horizontal surfaces weekly.

- Keep indoor humidity below 50 percent year-round.

- Open windows for an hour each day during dry seasons to improve ventilation.

- Use a HEPA air filter in the bedroom.

- Clean mold off shower curtains, bathroom and basement walls, and other surfaces with a solution of bleach, detergent, and water.

- Use a dehumidifier if your basement is damp or musty.

- Never allow smoking in the house.

"The air within homes and other buildings can be more seriously polluted than the outdoor air in even the largest and most industrialized cities."

—ENVIRONMENTAL PROTECTION AGENCY

95

Exercise Caution

At the gym, you're sharing equipment with some friends and mostly strangers, and germs with everyone. Along with the standard wipe-down, you can take important steps to cut down your risk of picking up an unwanted gym buddy:

- **Germs don't only lurk on handles and benches or in the locker room.** Today's high-tech fitness equipment is loaded with monitors and displays—unwitting places where bacteria can be harbored. One drop of spit can carry 100 million bacteria, and these monitors and displays are within the direct line of fire of someone's spit. Rhinovirus (which causes the common cold) and strep (which causes bronchitis or strep throat) have the run of equipment monitors and displays. Do not rest your towel or your reading material on these monitors and displays even though they're just the right size and place to do so.

- **Launder your gym towel daily.** Infectious bacteria and fungi (like the one that causes athlete's foot) breed on reused towels. Each time you towel off, you rub bacteria from your skin onto the towel. Seven days of continuous use of a towel is long enough for it to accumulate enough organic material to form a barrier that protects the bacteria, enabling the germs to multiply and invade.

- **Take a long shower after a workout, and disinfect and cover all cuts and abrasions that happen during a workout.** Methicillin-resistant *Staphylococcus aureus* (MRSA) is a superbug that can enter the bloodstream with deadly consequences. It is highly contagious and easily spreads through indirect contact by touching objects that have been contaminated by someone with MRSA.

- **Cut down on carbs and sweets.** Carbohydrates and sweets—including sugars in sports drinks—are foods that feed bacteria in the intestinal tract. If your gastrointestinal system is even a bit out of kilter ("intestinal dysbiosis"), and you exercise (which exhausts your body temporarily), carbs and sweets will serve to fuel the bad bacteria in the gut to multiply.

Find a personal trainer specializing in anti-aging sports medicine by contacting the American College of Anti-Aging Sportsmedicine Professionals (ACASP). Call 773-528-4333 or e-mail sports@worldhealth.net.

96

Create Your Sleep Haven

A sleep debt is the accumulated amount of lost sleep over time. Those who need seven hours of sleep a night, can, over a week, amass a sleep debt of seven hours if they get only six hours of sleep nightly. A sleep debt robs us of quality of life, deteriorating our physical and cognitive acuity slowly until we are overwhelmed by powerful and sudden sleepiness. The nationwide sleep debt, resulting in fatigue, has been reported to cost the American economy about $120 million annually in health expenditures, lost worker productivity, and property destruction.

Today, Americans are sleeping a full hour a day less than our ancestors did at the turn of the century. If you are fatigued or depressed, and have trouble thinking, reacting, and staying alert, you may very well have a sleep debt. Here are some ways to improve your odds of getting a good night's sleep:

- **Keep the sleeping room cool.** Lowering the temperature helps your body cool down, which can help to trigger sleep onset.

- **Keep the sleeping room dark.** Light is the most powerful time cue for humans; even low ambient light (such as that of a nightlight) alters the sleep-wake cycle by way of the pineal gland, which is a light-sensitive organ that detects light even if the eyes are closed.

- **Keep the sleeping room quiet.** If you cannot keep sound to an absolute minimum, use a fan, air cleaner, or other source of "white noise" to drown out discernable noise.

"American adults are sleeping 6.8 hours a night on weekdays and 7.4 hours a night on weekends."

—NATIONAL SLEEP FOUNDATION, 2005 SLEEP IN AMERICA POLL

97

Be a Social Butterfly

Social and productive activities provide equivalent advantages to staying alive as do physical fitness activities. Harvard Medical School researchers found that people with a chronic medical condition that makes physical exertion difficult may greatly benefit from participating in social activities.

Spend an afternoon tea with your friends, play bridge on Friday night, or have an impromptu get-together with neighbors. When you spend quality time with those who share your interests, you establish the basis for a social network that helps you to maintain a positive outlook on life.

> *"Let your life lightly dance on the edges of time*
> *like dew on the tip of a leaf."*
> —RABINDRANATH TAGORE, BENGALI POET,
> PLAYWRIGHT, AND NOVELIST

98

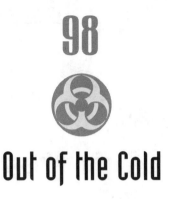

Out of the Cold

A 2005 study by researchers at the Federal Research Centre of Nutrition and Food in Germany found that those men and women who took daily vitamins and minerals with probiotics (bacteria that can activate the immune system, particularly T cells) for at least three months reported reduced cold symptoms compared with those suffered by people who took only vitamins and minerals. The men and women taking a combination of vitamins, minerals, and probiotics experienced the following:

- Colds that lasted almost two days less than the average of nine days.

- Less time with a fever, reduced to six hours, rather than the average of twenty-four hours.

- Less severe headaches, coughing, and sneezing.

Probiotic bacteria, in the form of *Lactobacillus* and *Bifidobacterium* strains, are found in respectable amounts in yogurt. They are also available, in higher doses, in dietary supplement form (freeze-dried powders, capsules, and wafers are preferable over liquid supplements, which are highly perishable). Look for probiotic supplements with the highest "colony forming units" per dose. Because bacteria counts drop as the product ages, mind the expiration date. Take probiotic supplements on an empty stomach.

"In the course of a year, people in the United States suffer 1 billion colds."

—U.S. National Institute of Allergy and Infectious Diseases

99

For Best Rest

We spend just about a third of our days sleeping, so it is important that the air in your bedroom be as pristine as possible. Here are some tips to minimize bedroom allergens:

- Vacuum often with a HEPA (high-efficiency particulate air) filter vacuum, which prevents dust particles from recirculating.

- Wash bedding weekly in hot water (130°F) and dry in a hot dryer.

- Replace pillows and mattresses made of natural materials like down and cotton with pillows and mattresses made of synthetic fibers.

- Encase mattresses and pillows in dust mite–proof covers. Wash blankets and pillowcases that aren't encased once a week in hot water.

- Do not allow pets into the bedroom. A study by Dr. Shepard of the Mayo Clinic Sleep Disorders Center reported that 53 percent of pet owners permitting the animal in the sleeping room had disrupted sleep every night. Pet allergies can also contribute to problems breathing during sleep.

- Leave dust-prone plants, knickknacks, and fuzzy stuffed toys out of the bedroom.

"The indoor environment [as compared to the outdoors] has higher contaminant levels and provides more immediate and prolonged exposure to pollutants."

—BATTELLE MEMORIAL INSTITUTE

100

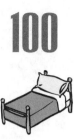

For Sleep, Less Is More

Minimize your odds of experiencing poor sleep by doing the following:

- Reduce sources of electromagnetic fields (EMFs), waves of electric and magnetic energies that are produced by electronic and electrical equipment. They can affect brainwaves so as to alter mental acuity and change mood and sleep patterns. EMFs are produced by electric clocks and clock radios, televisions and computers, cellular phones and cordless phones, lamps, and ionization–type smoke and carbon monoxide detectors. Keep these items at least 15 feet (4.6 meters) away from the bed.

- Reduce chemical irritants that may cause breathing difficulties, which can interfere with getting to sleep or getting a continuous night's sleep, by doing the following:

  - Remove home furnishings made with synthetics and those that are chemically treated (carpeting, furniture, draperies).

  - Do not bring freshly dry-cleaned clothes (high in vapors of the solvents used in the cleaning process) into the bedroom until aired out in a separate room for several days. Close the closet door before going to sleep.

  - Use natural, untreated cotton or silk sheets. Avoid "permanent press" sheets as these are treated with chemicals (most notably, formaldehyde).

"Go confidently in the direction of your dreams.
Live the life you have imagined."

—Henry David Thoreau, American author

101

Flush with Food

Thanks to today's contemporary lifestyle of fast foods, 24/7/365 accessibility, and the growing pressures of our professional and personal lives, we have become a population of toxemics. "Toxemia" is the medical term that defines a condition in which our bodies accumulate poisonous substances to such a point that levels exceed the ability of our body systems to cleanse them away. Medical conditions associated with toxemia include:

- Hepatitis A, B, C, D, E, F, and G

- Liver damage, including cirrhosis

- Diarrhea

- Constipation

- Irritable bowel syndrome

- Leaky gut syndrome

Include fiber in your daily diet, because fiber can promote the digestive and elimination processes to help your body get rid of toxins (see Tip 42).

The New Anti-Aging Revolution: Stopping the Clock for a Younger, Sexier, Happier You! by Ronald Klatz and Robert Goldman (Basic Health Publications, 2003) shares insights on preventive tactics that may promote longevity.

102

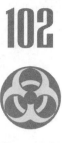

A Touchy Situation

In 2005, the American Society for Microbiology reported that while 91 percent of American adults say they always wash their hands after using public restrooms, in actuality only 83 percent did so. Women were more likely to wash their hands (90 percent) compared with men (75 percent). The same survey also revealed these other lackluster hand-washing habits:

- Only 21 percent of men and women say they always wash their hands after handling money.

- Only 24 percent of men and 39 percent of women say they always wash their hands after coughing or sneezing.

The technique for proper hand washing per the U.S. Centers for Disease Control and Prevention involves these steps:

1. Wet your hands and apply liquid or clean bar soap. Place the bar soap on a rack that allows it to drain.

2. Scrub all surfaces—including wrists, palms, backs of hands, fingers, under the fingernails, and between fingers. Rub your hands vigorously together for ten to fifteen seconds.

3. Rinse well with warm water.

4. Dry hands with a clean or disposable towel. Pat the skin rather than rubbing to avoid chapping or cracking.

"Washing your hands . . . costs less than a penny and is a way of prevention that can save you a $50 visit to the doctor."

—U.S. National Center for Infectious Diseases

103

Is the Bed to Blame?

The bed is not merely a home furnishing, it is an integral part of your sleep environment. Be sure to consider the following:

- If you share a bed, you and your partner may sleep best in a king-size bed, particularly if you or your bed partner is prone to tossing and turning or has restless leg syndrome. Two adults in a double- or queen-size bed only have as much horizontal space as a baby does in a crib!

- A properly selected and maintained mattress provides positive resistance to the sleeper's body weight. Goldilocks was right:
  - A mattress that is too firm will not provide even body support, tending instead to support only at the body's heaviest parts (shoulders and hips).
  - A mattress that is too soft will not keep the spine in proper alignment with the rest of the body. As a result, your muscles will work throughout the night to straighten the spine, leading to aches and pains in the morning.

- Rotate your mattress and turn it over every two to three months to reduce sags, imprints, bumps, and valleys.

- The foundation part of the bed, the box spring, extends the life of the mattress. It absorbs the major portion of the stress and weight placed on the sleep surface.

"Only half of adults can say they get a good night's sleep a few nights/week or more. Fifty percent (50%) report feeling tired, fatigued, or not up to par during wake time at least one day a week."
—National Sleep Foundation, 2005 Sleep in America poll

104

Keep Stress in Check

The hormone cortisol is produced during times of stress by the adrenal glands, which are located atop the kidneys. You can reduce cortisol production by restoring adrenal balance, including by boosting the adrenal gland production of DHEA (see Tip 46). Also do the following:

- **Go outdoors**—A lack of natural light causes seasonal depression and may lead to an imbalance in adrenal function. Go outside for at least one hour each day, making sure to splash on the sunscreen that's appropriate for your skin protection needs.

- **Go whole**—Eat a whole foods diet. Minimize (preferably, eliminate) caffeine, sugar, and alcohol—substances that elevate adrenal function.

- **Supplement the adrenals**—Consider taking a daily nutritional supplement of DHEA or Siberian ginseng, which contains a compound that the body uses to manufacture pregnenolone, the precursor to DHEA. Consult an anti-aging physician to determine the best dose for you.

- **Identify possible food allergies**—With the help of an anti-aging physician, find food triggers of stress and develop a proper food rotation diet to keep the physical demands on the adrenal glands to a minimum.

Visit the World Health Network at www.worldhealth.net, the website of the A4M, and use the interactive directory to locate a qualified anti-aging physician and/or clinic in your geographic area.

105

Not So Fine

Fine particles—particulate matter in the air measuring less than 2.5 microns in diameter—can cause serious health problems. According to the American Lung Association, "tens of thousands of premature deaths each year are attributed to fine particle air pollution," microscopic substances such as acid aerosols, organic chemicals, metals, and carbon soot.

Long-term studies have repeatedly shown that people living in areas with high fine particle concentration may have their lives shortened by one to two years on average (compared with those living in cleaner locations).

To limit your exposure to fine particle air pollution, be sure to:

- **Stay in an indoor environment where the air is filtered or air-conditioned.** You can build an inexpensive air purifier by taping a micropore HEPA air conditioner filter over a large box fan.

- **Do not exercise outdoors when particulate levels are high.** Never exercise near high-traffic areas.

- **Drink plenty of fluids.** See Tip 36.

- **Take a cool shower or bath.** This removes superficial particulate matter from your skin.

In the United States, the Air Quality Index (AQI) is the standard system that state and local air pollution control programs use to notify the public about levels of air pollution. The U.S. Environmental Protection Agency (EPA) posts the daily AQI at www.epa.gov/airnow.

106

Protective Pets

Children in families with cats or dogs have fewer pet allergies than new pet owners or those who had only been exposed earlier in life.

A 2005 study by researchers at the Central Hospital of Norrbotten in Sweden, which tracked 2,454 children for four years, found that in all cases where allergies were not a result of genetics, exposure to animal allergens protected boys and girls from developing allergies. A previous study, conducted by researchers at the Institute for Social Pediatrics and Adolescent Medicine in Germany found that children who were continually exposed to pets (in this study, cats) were 67 percent less likely than other kids to develop asthma and 45 percent less likely to develop hay fever.

"A faithful friend is the medicine of life."

—APOCRYPHA

107

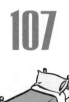

Foil the Common Sleep Robbers

If you experience trouble falling asleep, or staying asleep, consider the following:

- An irregular or inconsistent schedule of being awake/asleep sets the biological stage for poor sleep. Set a regular schedule, particularly for the time at which you get up every day.

- Avoid caffeine (commonly found in soda, soft drinks, coffee, and tea), which is a stimulant, for six hours before bedtime, longer if you know this substance gives you trouble sleeping. Also avoid hidden sources of caffeine, such as chocolate and some over-the-counter pain and cold remedies.

- Avoid nicotine, which is also a stimulant, from cigarettes and nicotine-replacement products, for at least six hours before bedtime.

- Avoid drinking alcohol after dinnertime. While a drink may help you fall asleep, it will probably cause you to awaken in the middle of the night.

- If you are on any prescription or over-the-counter medications, find out from your doctor or pharmacist if any of them could be keeping you awake or causing you to not get a refreshing sleep.

"Seventy-eight percent (78 percent) of Americans drink at least one cup or can of a caffeinated beverage daily (soda, soft drinks, coffee, or tea)."
—NATIONAL SLEEP FOUNDATION, 2005 SLEEP IN AMERICA POLL

108

Men Be Wary of Plastics

Low levels of a chemical found in plastic containers and tin cans increases the risk of prostate abnormalities, reports a 2005 study conducted at the University of South Dakota School of Medicine. While the study was conducted on mice, researchers warn the same findings could hold true for men, because exposure levels by the lab animals in the study were far lower than that of a human baby.

Blood levels of the compound bisphenol A at levels well below thresholds deemed safe by the U.S. Environmental Protection Agency area were found to cause malformations of the prostates of developing animals, and these malformations were suspected to predispose these animals to prostate cancer as adults. The study also found that male mouse fetuses exposed to bisphenol A developed abnormally enlarged prostate ducts, putting them at risk for a condition similar to benign prostate hypertrophy (BPH).

"Prostate cancer is the most common form of cancer among men in the United States, other than skin cancer. In 2004, approximately 230,110 new cases of prostate cancer will be diagnosed and 29,900 men will die of the disease."

—U.S. CENTERS FOR DISEASE CONTROL AND PREVENTION

109

Have a Plan

Before a natural disaster strikes, create your Emergency Plan. It should include the following features:

- **Call for the Basics:** Contact your State Emergency Management Office to find out:
  - What kinds of natural disasters might happen in your area.
  - What type of warning system(s) are in place.
  - What your local evacuation route options are.
  - What special help would be available for the elderly or disabled.
  - Also, find out from your workplace, your partner's workplace, and your children's school or daycare, what their Emergency Plans are.

- **Create your Plan:**
  - Meet with your family members to brief them on what you found. Collect their questions and be sure to incorporate the answers into your plan.
  - Be familiar with (and make sure all adults in the home are familiar with) switches to turn off water, gas, and electricity that supply the house.
  - Teach children how and when to call 911, police, and fire departments.

- Establish evacuation routes from your home and a meeting place a safe distance from your home. Practice your evacuation at least twice a year.

- Post emergency telephone numbers near each phone.

- Keep family records and important documents in a safety deposit box at a bank.

- Pick one out-of-state and one local friend or relative for family members to contact if separated during a disaster.

- Be sure to include instructions to address elderly or disabled family members if they reside in your home.

• Have a Disaster Supplies Kit always at-the-ready (see Tip 112).

"In fair weather prepare for foul."
—THOMAS FULLER,
ENGLISH CHURCHMAN AND HISTORIAN

110

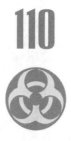

Kitchen Germ-ination

The kitchen can be a germination ground that breeds bacteria that may contaminate food and can then get us sick. There are about 76 million cases of food-borne illnesses a year, and most of them occur from bugs in our very own homes. While no kitchen will ever be germ-free, here are some tips that can help reduce the bacteria that might transfer into food:

- Wash your hands (see Tip 102) before beginning to prepare food. Wash them again after you touch raw meat, fish, or vegetables, and between touching these different foods (to reduce cross-contamination).

- Microwave kitchen sponges on high for one minute until steaming, every day.

- Launder or microwave dishcloths regularly, three or more times a week.

- Clean the kitchen sink drain, disposal, and connecting pipe once a week. Sanitize them by pouring down the sink a solution of 1 teaspoon (5 milliliters) of chlorine bleach in 1 quart (about 1 liter) of water or a solution of commercial kitchen cleaning agent prepared according to product directions. Food particles get trapped in the drain and disposal and, along with the moistness, create an ideal environment for bacterial growth.

"An estimated 76 million cases of food-borne disease occur each year in the United States. Serious cases can result in 325,000 hospitalizations and 5,000 deaths annually."

—U.S. CENTERS FOR DISEASE CONTROL AND PREVENTION

111

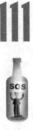

Work Can Indeed Be Toxic

In a study by researchers at Buckinghamshire Chilterns University College, those subjects who worked for a boss they considered to be unfair experienced a 15 mm Hg increase in their systolic pressure and a 7 mm Hg increase in their diastolic pressure (compared with days on which they worked for a boss they considered as more favorable). A rise of just 10 mm Hg systolic pressure and/or 5 mm Hg diastolic pressure is associated with a 16 percent higher risk of heart disease and 38 percent increased risk of stroke.

Work with your boss to create a fair and considerate working environment, which will not only reduce the risks to your health, but will promote productivity and improve workplace morale to the benefit of management.

"There are two kinds of people, those who do the work and those who take the credit. Try to be in the first group; there is less competition there."

—INDIRA GANDHI, INDIAN POLITICAL LEADER

112

Use in Case of Emergency

The American Red Cross recommends several basics you should stock for your home in the case of an emergency. Keep the items that you would most likely need during an evacuation in an easy-to-carry container (such as a covered trash container, a camping backpack, or a duffle bag) that is kept in a readily accessible location (the guest closet or garage, for example).

Your Disaster Supplies Kit should include:

- **Water**—One gallon of water per person per day; keep at least a seven-day supply of water per person.

- **Food**—A seven-day supply of nonperishable food.

- **First-aid supplies**—See the website below for an example of what's included in a first-aid kit.

- **Medications for health conditions**

- **Clothing**

- **Bedding**

- **Tools and emergency supplies**

- **Special items necessary for infants and elderly or disabled persons**

- **Copies of key family documents**—Birth certificates, marriage certificates, passports, drivers licenses, banking and credit card account numbers, insurance policies, health records, household inventory lists; see the website below for a more thorough list.

 Visit the American Red Cross website, at www.redcross.org, to learn more about how to prepare for disasters.

113

Procrastination Payoff

Researchers at Kinston University in the United Kingdom reported in 2005 that an unmade bed, while unattractive to the eyes, is unappealing to dust mites—tiny bugs, shorter than 1 mm long—that feed on shed human skin cells and produce excretions that, when inhaled by people, can cause allergic reactions and asthma. According to the team, the average bed can house as many as 1.5 million dust mites. When a bed is made immediately or shortly after people get out of it, moisture can become trapped in the sheets and mattress, creating a haven for the mites. Moisture is minimized in unmade beds, and as a result, the mites will be more likely to dehydrate and die than feast and multiply.

Infection Protection: How to Fight the Germs That Make You Sick by Ronald Klatz and Robert Goldman (HarperCollins, 2002) shares insights on how to minimize germs in everyday settings.

114

Green Groceries

The United Nations estimates that at least 4 million people worldwide have Parkinson's disease (PD), a type of motor system disorder that is marked by tremor, rigidity, slowness of movement, and postural instability.

Environmental exposures increase a person's risk of developing PD. Even when genes are a factor in the disease, as with many familial cases, exposure to toxins or other environmental factors may influence when symptoms of the disease appear and/or how the disease progresses. Pesticides and fungicides produce free radicals that cause cellular oxidative stress, one of the main causes of degeneration of brain cells. In a 2005 study by University of Rochester researchers, pesticides and fungicides were found to remain on produce for more than three weeks and persisted even after washing.

Whenever possible, purchase locally grown fruits and vegetables and encourage your grocer to provide produce that is free of pesticides and fungicides.

The New Anti-Aging Revolution: Stopping the Clock for a Younger, Sexier, Happier You! by Ronald Klatz and Robert Goldman (Basic Health Publications, 2003) shares insights on preventive tactics that may promote longevity.

115

Emergency Water Disinfection

In the event of a natural disaster, which may compromise your access to water from your tap or bottle source, follow these techniques to purify water for drinking:

- **Boiling:** Vigorously, for ten minutes

- **Bleaching:** Add 10–20 drops of household bleach per gallon of water, mix well, and let stand for thirty minutes. A slight smell or taste of chlorine indicates water is good to drink. (Note: do not use scented or color-safe bleaches, or ones with added cleaners.)

- **Tablets:** Commercially available purification tablets

- **Solar disinfection, known as SODIS:** A new technique developed by researchers at the Swiss Federal Institute for Environmental Science and Technology. Clear plastic bottles are filled with water and left in the sun. The heat warms the water and the combination of warm water and ultraviolet radiation kills most microorganisms. The Institute's tests showed that 99.9 percent of the *E. coli* bacteria in a sample of contaminated water were killed when the sun heated the water beyond 122°F (50°C). At that temperature, disinfection takes about an hour, but placing a corrugated metal sheet under the bottle can shorten the time. Additional tests demonstrate SODIS as an effective approach for killing the cholera bacteria, *Vibrio cholerae,* and that it could inactivate parasites including the diarrhea-causing *Cryptosporidium.*

"One of the tests of leadership is the ability to recognize a problem before it becomes an emergency."

—Arnold Glasgow, political leader

116

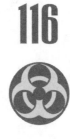

Watch Your Mouth

The mouth can harbor 500 different kinds of microorganisms, which readily and rapidly reproduce in the warm, dark, moist environment and can enter the body through the airways and digestive pathways. Dental problems have been linked to the following diseases:

- **Heart disease**—Bacteria in the mouth can enter the bloodstream and may deposit into the vessels that supply the heart. A University of North Carolina study found that 85 percent of heart attack victims had severe gum disease.

- **Stroke**—Studies have found that people with severe gum disease have twice the risk of stroke (compared with people who have good oral health).

- **Diabetes**—Diabetics with gum disease are three times more likely to have heart attacks (compared with diabetics without).

- **Pneumonia**—A University of Buffalo research study found that germs found in dental plaque can cause pneumonia, as respiratory pathogens in the plaque can readily be inhaled into the lungs.

Here are some ways to stop deadly germs from multiplying and spreading from your mouth:

- Eat a balanced and nutritional diet.
- Limit sugar consumption.
- Brush and floss twice a day.
- Visit the dentist regularly for preventive checkups and cleanings.

"Most adults show signs of gum disease. Severe gum disease affects about 14 percent of adults aged 45 to 54 years."

—U.S. CENTERS FOR DISEASE CONTROL AND PREVENTION

117

A Healthy Gum-ption

Enjoy these foods and beverages that have been shown to promote good oral health:

- **Green tea**—University of Illinois–Chicago researchers found that drinking green tea reduced the number of bacteria in the mouth that cause bad breath. In a separate study, Pace University scientists found that flavorids, a compound in green tea, work with the germ killers in toothpaste and mouthwash, boosting their effectiveness at warding off viruses and preventing cavities.

- **Black tea**—A study by the Vivekananda Institute in India reported in 2005 that people who drank black tea for one year had a reduced risk of developing oral cancer.

- **Cranberry juice**—Researchers at the University of Rochester have shown that cranberry juice helps to stop bacteria from sticking to teeth, thereby preventing the formation of plaque (the cause of tooth decay and gum disease). Separate research by a team at University of Illinois–Chicago found that cranberry juice interfered with the viability and growth of oral pathogens.

- **Raisins**—In 2005, University of Illinois–Chicago researchers found that two compounds in raisins were successful in fighting bacteria in the mouth that cause cavities and gum disease.

"In the United States, one in seven adults aged 35 to 44 years has gum disease; this increases to one in every four adults aged 65 years and older."

—U.S. Centers for Disease Control and Prevention

118

Supplemental Sleep

Many of us are not getting the necessary amount or quality of sleep we need each night in order to function at our best the next day (see Tip 96). Napping cannot necessarily make up for inadequate or poor-quality nighttime sleep, but taking a short nap (20–30 minutes) does have its benefits. According to the U.S. National Sleep Foundation:

- Naps can restore alertness, enhance performance, and reduce mistakes and accidents. A study by the U.S. National Aeronautics and Space Administration (NASA) on sleepy military pilots and astronauts found that a forty-minute nap improved performance by 34 percent and alertness by 100 percent.

- Naps can increase alertness in the period directly following the nap and may extend alertness a few hours later in the day.

- Scheduled napping has also been prescribed for those who are affected by narcolepsy.

- Napping has psychological benefits. A nap can be a pleasant luxury, a mini vacation. It can provide an easy way to get some relaxation and rejuvenation.

"Fifty-five percent (55 percent) of Americans take, on average, at least one nap during the week."
—NATIONAL SLEEP FOUNDATION, 2005 SLEEP IN AMERICA POLL

119

Future Financial Fitness

Saving $100 a month, and presuming a federal tax rate of 25 percent and state tax rate of 6 percent, after twenty years, your savings will be valued at $128,229.71 ($69,730.59 after adjusting for a 3 percent inflation rate). It would take forty-five years and six months for that monthly $100 to reach $1 million (before adjusting for inflation).

A wiser investment: Each payday, pay yourself in the form of a zero coupon bond, which accrues compounded interest tax-free. You'll become a millionaire faster, and the sooner you start, the more you will amass.

*"The way money goes so fast these days,
they should paint racing stripes on it."*

—MARK RUSSELL, AMERICAN COMEDIAN,
PIANIST, AND SINGER

120

The New Circle of Life

A 2005 study by Merrill Lynch found that 77 percent of men and women ages forty to fifty-eight plan to work in retirement. Some of these people will become consultants in the industry in which they worked all their lives, while others will embark on a completely new career. A retirement job can boost your nest egg significantly.

Assuming you retire at age sixty-five, work two days a week earning 40 percent of what you earned before retiring, you can increase your savings by up to 30 percent over a five-year period. Working during retirement also helps to maintain a social network, which has been found to be key in maintaining a meaningful life.

> *"Retirement at sixty-five is ridiculous.*
> *When I was sixty-five I still had pimples."*
>
> —GEORGE BURNS, AMERICAN COMEDIAN AND ACTOR

121

Share the Health

The American Academy of Anti-Aging Medicine (A4M) is the leading worldwide medical organization dedicated to the advancement of technology to detect, prevent, and treat age-related disease and to promote research into methods to retard and optimize the human aging process. As a United States federally registered non-profit medical organization, A4M is also dedicated to educating physicians, scientists, and members of the public on anti-aging issues. A4M believes that the disabilities associated with normal aging are caused by physiological dysfunction, which in many cases are ameliorable to medical treatment, such that the human life span can be increased, and the quality of one's life improved as one grows chronologically older.

Through its Internet presence (www.worldhealth.net), publications, and scientific education programs, A4M shares information concerning innovative science and research as well as treatment modalities designed to prolong the healthy human life span.

We commend you on taking the time to read this book. We hope that you have learned new ways to help you live a long and healthy life. We encourage you to share the health by passing along this book to family members or friends, so they may do the same.

"The first wealth is health."

—RALPH WALDO EMERSON, AMERICAN AUTHOR,
POET, AND PHILOSOPHER

Conclusion
Toward Practical Immortality

In *121 Ways to Live to 121 Years . . . and More!* we share with you practical tips based on today's knowledge that can help you live a long and healthy life.

It is our position that we need only bridge the gap between the medical knowledge of today and the medical knowledge that we will have in our grasp by 2029. Since medical knowledge doubles every three and a half years or less, by 2029 we will know at least 256 times more than we know today! As a result, it is not impracticable nor improbable to expect that humankind will reach the point where we'll know how to substantially slow or perhaps even stop aging, and even eventually reset the clock mechanism of life itself.

By the year 2029, we anticipate that science will accomplish practical immortality: healthy human life spans of 150 years and beyond.

We may consider the years from 2006 through 2029 collectively as a Bridge to Practical Immortality, during which science will amass key knowledge in biomedical technologies that will enable 150+ year-long life spans.

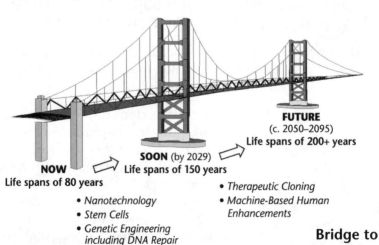

FUTURE
(c. 2050–2095)
Life spans of 200+ years

SOON (by 2029)
Life spans of 150 years

NOW
Life spans of 80 years

- *Nanotechnology*
- *Stem Cells*
- *Genetic Engineering including DNA Repair*
- *Artificial Organs*

- *Therapeutic Cloning*
- *Machine-Based Human Enhancements*

Bridge to Practical Immortality

In the meantime, we can rely on the expertise and experience of anti-aging physicians to usher us across the Bridge to Practical Immortality, deploying the twelve tenets of anti-aging medicine:

1. Anti-aging endocrinology and hormone-replacement therapy
2. Antioxidant analysis and optimized supplementation
3. Maximized immune function
4. Detoxification
5. Cardiovascular protection
6. Cognitive function assessment and repair
7. Metabolic and DNA repair
8. Skin de-aging and repair
9. Lifestyle modification
10. Musculoskeletal rehabilitation-sports medicine-conditioning
11. Biomarkers of aging assessment
12. Prospective advanced diagnostics

With the guidance of a qualified anti-aging physician, you can start your anti-aging transformation today.

JOIN THESE NEW A4M PROJECTS AND HELP REWRITE THE FUTURE OF HUMAN AGING

A4M invites you to join us in two of our primary project initiatives that we submit are the natural and next progressions to advance the anti-aging medical movement, namely:

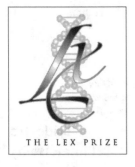

THE LEX PRIZE

The LEx (Life Extension) Prize, a $1 million cash prize to be awarded to the first researcher(s) or scientist(s) who accomplish the goal of reliably demonstrating the reversal or halting of the aging process in humans, as defined by The LEx Prize Criteria. The winning scientists or researchers must demonstrate that the therapeutic program has reduced select, key objective biomarkers of aging in ten human subjects (ages 70 years or more), by twenty years each. Details, including a list of the specific LEx Prize biomarkers, as well as application and procedure information, are online at www.a4minfo.net/lexprize.

We gratefully acknowledge the generous contributions of prominent physicians, scientists, and patrons of the anti-aging medical movement. Leading individual LEx Prize pledges received to date include:

- $100,000 from A4M Chairman Robert Goldman, M.D., Ph.D., D.O., F.A.A.S.P.

- $100,000 from A4M President Ronald Klatz, M.D., D.O.

- $100,000 from Sam Weaver, Ph.D. and Carol Weaver, Ed.D.

- $25,000 from Eric Braverman, M.D.

- $25,000 from Ron Rothenberg, M.D.

- $25,000 from Mark Gordon, M.D.

- $10,000 from Nick Delgado, Ph.D

With your support, we can make the LEx Prize a success, and the reversal of aging a reality. Direct questions on this project to: lexprize@a4minfo.net.

Critical to the advancement of the anti-aging medical movement worldwide is the creation of **The World Center for Anti-Aging Medicine**, a Center of Excellence at which medical innovations relating to enhancement and/or extension of the healthy human life span are fostered. The World Center merges clinical and research objectives in an innovative vision of the future of medicine. Researchers yielding discoveries that will revolutionize the very early detection, treatment, and rejuvenation of aging-related disorders will work alongside clinicians delivering multi-therapeutic interventions designed to slow, stop, and/or reverse the process of human aging. The World Center is a state-of-the-art facility at which the greatest contemporary scientific minds will conduct studies to discover the secrets of aging and devise novel, effective interventions to prolong quality and quantity of life. Details on the World Center for Anti-Aging Medicine are online at www.a4minfo. net/center.

The World Center for Anti-Aging Medicine is projected to need $30 million in initial funding, of which the A4M has already secured private commitments totaling $2 million. For the shortfall, the A4M seeks angel benefactors who share our vision to realize anti-aging breakthroughs for the benefit of humanity. The business plan is largely ready for implementation, as the A4M has defined all the start-up and ongoing costs necessary for the project. With your support, the vision of a Center of Excellence in Anti-Aging Medicine can be realized.

This is a once-in-a-lifetime opportunity to achieve personal and historic status as a patron of the new science of anti-aging medicine. The World Center for Anti-Aging Medicine will revolutionize the practice of medicine and enhance our lives and those of generations to follow.

Direct questions on this project to center@a4minfo.net.

LEXMD.com

Physicians' picks of the "best of the best" products from the new science of anti-aging medicine.

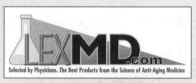

Selected by Physicians. The Best Products from the Science of Anti-Aging Medicine

Individually reviewed and selected by a panel of top physicians and scientists from the anti-aging medical specialty, all products offered at www.LEXMD.com are:

• Supported by reliable independent scientific studies

• Manufactured from the highest quality ingredients

• Offer the best value

In addition, all products at www.lexmd.com are backed by a 100% absolute satisfaction, no-hassle, money-back guarantee.

www.LEXMD.com is the intelligent place to shop online for all your nutritional medicine and anti-aging therapeutics needs.

Recommended Resources

The American Academy of Anti-Aging Medicine (A4M)

Educational website: *www.worldhealth.net*

A4M is the world's leading professional organization dedicated to advancing research and clinical pursuits that enhance the quality, and extend the quantity, of the human life span. A registered 501(c)3 nonprofit organization, the A4M is comprised of members totaling 18,500 and representing eighty-five nations worldwide. Join A4M to gain first access to information about the very latest breakthroughs that may help you live a longer, healthier life. Membership includes:

- **Complimentary subscription to our award-winning journal,** *Anti-Aging Medical News*

- **Networking at A4M-Sponsored Events:** A4M co-sponsors scientific educational programs that are recognized by the Accreditation Council for Continuing Medical Education (ACCME). Meet thousands of doctors, guest speakers, exhibitors, and key members of the industry.

- **Discounts on A4M academic publications and multimedia products:** Learn anti-aging from the organization that created the anti-aging specialty. Choose from an extensive array of books, DVDs, and CDs.

The World Health Network ▪ www.worldhealth.net

The educational website of the A4M, the World Health Network is the Internet's leading anti-aging portal. It receives more than 20 million hits a month and holds top-ranked listings on Yahoo!, Google, and MSN. The World Health Network's online interactive directory assists more than 20,000 people a month in finding a qualified anti-aging doctor or clinic in their geographic area.

BioTech e-Newsletter—FREE! ($149 value)

The online newsletter of the World Health Network, the BioTech e-Newsletter reports from medical correspondents at twenty-six universities and medical research centers and covers the latest and most promising advances in medicine that relate to the early detection, treatment, prevention, and reversal of age-related conditions in medicine that appear in more than 100 scientific publications and news services weekly.

The BioTech e-Newsletter is a FREE service of the World Health Network: go to www.worldhealth.net and subscribe today.

SUGGESTED ADDITIONAL READING

The New Anti-Aging Revolution: Stopping the Clock for a Younger, Sexier, Happier You!, by Dr. Ronald Klatz and Dr. Robert Goldman (Basic Health Publications, Inc., 2003)

Infection Protection: How to Fight the Germs That Make You Sick, by Dr. Ronald Klatz and Dr. Robert Goldman (HarperCollins, 2002)

Brain Fitness: Anti-Aging Strategies for Achieving Super Mind Power, by Dr. Robert Goldman with Dr. Ronald Klatz and Lisa Berger (Mainstreet Books, 1999)

> **Visit the A4M Bookstore**
> **at the World Health Network,**
> **www.worldhealth.net**

Index

About the Authors

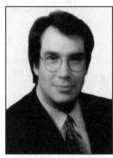

Dr. Ronald Klatz, who coined the term "anti-aging medicine," is recognized as a leading authority in the new clinical science of anti-aging medicine. Since 1981, Dr. Klatz has been integral in the pioneering exploration of new therapies for the treatment and prevention of age-related degenerative diseases. He is the physician founder and president of the American Academy of Anti-Aging Medicine Inc. (A4M), a nonprofit medical organization dedicated to the advancement of technology to detect, prevent, and treat age-related disease and to promote research into methods to retard and optimize the human aging process. As a world-renowned expert in anti-aging medicine, Dr. Klatz is a popular lecturer at A4M sponsored/co-supported events in anti-aging medicine. He is instrumental in the continuing development of A4M's educational website, www.worldhealth.net, with an Internet audience exceeding 300,000 viewers, for which he serves as Senior Medical Editor.

Dr. Klatz oversees continuing medical education programs co-sponsored by A4M that are AMA/ACCME approved, for more than 30,000 physicians, health practitioners, and scientists from eighty-five countries worldwide each year. In addition, Dr. Klatz is Professor, Department of Internal Medicine at the University of Central America Health Sciences. Dr. Klatz is board certified in the specialties of family practice, sports medicine, and anti-aging medicine.

Dr. Klatz co-founded the National Academy of Sports Medicine, which provides medical specialty training in musculoskeletal rehabilitation, conditioning, physical fitness, and exercise to 35,000 healthcare professionals internationally. He was a founder and key patent developer for Organ Recovery Systems, a biomedical research company focusing on technologies for brain resuscitation, trauma and emergency medicine, organ transplant, and blood preservation.

Dr. Klatz is the inventor, developer, or administrator of numerous medical and scientific patents. In recognition of his pioneering medical breakthroughs, he was awarded the Gold Medal in Science for Brain Resuscitation Technology (1993) and the Grand Prize in Medicine for Brain Cooling Technology (1994). In addition, Dr. Klatz has been named as a Top 10 Medical Innovator in Biomedical Technology (1997) by the National Institute of Electromedical Information, and received the Ground Breaker Award in Health Care (1999) with Presidential Acknowledgment by William Jefferson Clinton from Transitional Services of New York.

The author of several nonfiction bestsellers, including *Grow Young with HGH* (HarperCollins, 1997), Dr. Klatz also has co-authored *The New Anti-Aging Revolution* (Basic Health Publications, 2003), *Infection Protection* (Harper Resource, 2002), *Ten Weeks to a Younger You* (Sports Tech Labs, 1999), *New Anti-Aging Secrets for Maximum Lifespan* (Sports Tech Labs, 1999), *Brain Fitness* (Bantam Doubleday Dell, 1999), *Hormones of Youth* (Sports Tech Labs, 1998), *Seven Anti-Aging Secrets* (Elite Sports Medicine, 1996), *Death in the Locker Room: Drugs & Sports* (Elite Sports Medicine, 1992), and *The E Factor* (William Morrow & Co., 1988).

Dr. Klatz has served as a contributor, editor, reviewer, and advisor to *Archives of Gerontology and Geriatrics*, *Journal of Gerontology*, *Osteopathic Annals Medical Journal*, *Patient Care Medical Journal*, *Total Health for Longevity*, and *50+ Plus* magazine. His columns on wellness and longevity have appeared in *Pioneer Press* (a division of Time-Life Inc.), *Townsend Letter for Doctors and Patients*, *Spa Management Journal*, *The Wellness Channel*, *Fitness & Longevity Digest*, *Alternative Medicine Digest*, *Nutritional Science News*, *Healing Retreats & Spas*, *Skin Inc.*, and *Longevity SA* (for which he had served as Senior Medical Editor).

Dr. Klatz has co-hosted the national Fox Network television series *Anti-Aging Update* and served as national advisor for Physician's Radio Network. He has appeared in interviews on *CNN*, *USA Today TV*, *ABC News*, *NBC News*, *CBS News*, *Good Morning America*, *The Today Show*, the *Oprah Winfrey Show*, *Extra Daily TV News* (partial list). Dr. Klatz has participated in articles appearing in *The New York Times*, *USA Today*, *Chicago Tribune*, *Newsweek*, *Harper's Bazaar*, *MacLean's* (Canada), *Forbes Magazine*, and *Investor's Business Daily* (partial list).

Dr. Klatz is highly regarded by scientific and academic colleagues for his continuing medical education lectures on the demographics of aging and the impact of biomedical technologies on longevity. His scientific articles have been published in *Resident and Staff Physician, British Journal of Sports Medicine, Medical Times/The Journal of Family Medicine, Osteopathic Annals,* and *American Medical Association News* (partial list).

Dr. Klatz is a graduate of Florida Technological University. He received the Doctor of Medicine (M.D.) Degree from the Central America Health Sciences University, School of Medicine, a government-sanctioned, Ministry of Health-approved, and World Health Organization–listed medical university. Dr. Klatz received his Doctor of Osteopathic Medicine and Surgery (D.O.) degree from the College of Osteopathic Medicine and Surgery (Des Moines, Iowa).

Dr. Klatz has held several distinguished teaching or research positions, at Tufts University, the University of Oklahoma School of Osteopathic Medicine, Des Moines University School of Medicine, and the Chicago College of Osteopathic Medicine.

A consultant to the biotechnology industry and a respected advisor to several members of the U.S. Congress and others on Capitol Hill, Dr. Klatz devotes much of his time to research and to the development of advanced biosciences for the benefit of humanity.

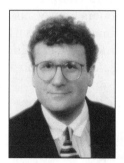

Dr. Robert Goldman has spearheaded the development of numerous international medical organizations and corporations. Dr. Goldman has served as a Senior Fellow at the Lincoln Filene Center, Tufts University, and as an Affiliate at the Philosophy of Education Research Center, Graduate School of Education, Harvard University. Dr. Goldman is Professor; Graduate School of Medicine, Swinburne University, Australia, and Clinical Consultant, Department of Obstetrics and Gynecology, Korea Medical University. He is also Professor, Department of Internal Medicine at the University of Central America Health Sciences, Department of Internal Medicine. Dr. Goldman is a Fellow of the American Academy of Sports Physicians and a Board Diplomat in Sports Medicine and Board Certified in Anti-Aging Medicine.

Dr. Goldman received his Bachelor of Science Degree (B.S.) from

Brooklyn College in New York, then conducted three years of independent research in steroid biochemistry and attended the State University of New York. He received the Doctor of Medicine (M.D.) Degree from the Central America Health Sciences University, School of Medicine in Belize, a government-sanctioned, Ministry of Health-approved, and World Health Organization–listed medical university. He received his Doctor of Osteopathic Medicine and Surgery (D.O.) degree from Chicago College of Osteopathic Medicine at Midwestern University. His Ph.D. work was in the field of androgenic anabolic steroid biochemistry.

He co-founded and serves as Chairman of the Board of Life Science Holdings, a biomedical research company which has had more than 150 medical patents under development in the areas of brain resuscitation, trauma and emergency medicine, organ transplant, and blood preservation technologies. He has overseen cooperative research agreement development programs in conjunction with such prominent institutions as the American National Red Cross, the U.S. National Aeronautics and Space Administration (NASA), the Department of Defense, and the FDA's Center for Devices & Radiological Health.

Dr. Goldman is the recipient of the Gold Medal for Science (1993), the Grand Prize for Medicine (1994), the Humanitarian Award (1995), and the Business Development Award (1996).

During the late 1990s, Dr. Goldman received honors from Minister of Sports and government health officials of numerous nations. In 2001, Excellency Juan Antonio Samaranch awarded Dr. Goldman the International Olympic Committee Tribute Diploma for contributions to the development of sport and Olympism.

In addition, Dr. Goldman is a black belt in karate, Chinese weapons expert, and world champion athlete with over twenty world strength records. He has also been listed in the *Guinness Book of World Records*. Some of his past performance records include 13,500 consecutive sit-ups and 321 consecutive handstand pushups.

Dr. Goldman was an All-College athlete in four sports, a three-time winner of the John F. Kennedy (JFK) Physical Fitness Award, was voted Athlete of the Year, was the recipient of the Champions Award, and was inducted into the World Hall of Fame of Physical Fitness. In 1995, Dr. Goldman was awarded the Healthy American Fitness Leader Award from the President's Council on Physical Fitness & Sports and U.S. Chamber of Commerce.

Dr. Goldman is Chairman of the International Medical Commission overseeing sports medicine committees in more than 176 nations. He has served as a Special Advisor to the President's Council on Physical Fitness & Sports. He is founder and international President Emeritus of the National Academy of Sports Medicine and the cofounder and chairman of the American Academy of Anti-Aging Medicine (A4M). Dr. Goldman visits an average of twenty countries annually to promote brain research and sports medicine programs.

World Records Held by Dr. Goldman

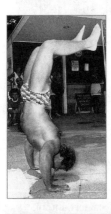

World Record:
321 Consecutive
Handstand Pushups

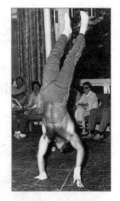

World Record:
50-Yard Handstand
Sprint Trial

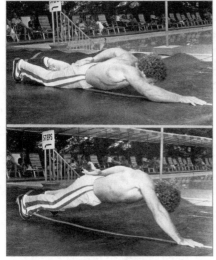

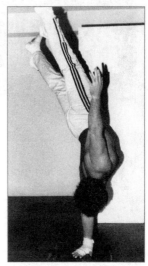

World Record: 161 Consecutive
Overhead Extension One-Arm Pushups

One-Arm Handstand
Pushup

Dr. Goldman, President's Council on Physical Fitness & Sports

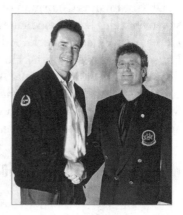

Dr. Goldman served as Special Advisor to the President's Council on Physical Fitness & Sports under Governor Schwarzenegger's Chairmanship of the Council.

Dr. Goldman (right) with friend Gov. Arnold Schwarzenegger.

Dr. Goldman, Recipient of the Gold Order of the International Federation of Body Builders (IFBB)

Dr. Robert Goldman, World Chairman IFBB Medical Commission, receives the IFBB's highest award—the IFBB Gold Order—at the World Championships in Shanghai, China, in 2005.

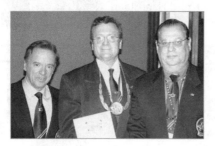

Dr. Goldman (center), shown here with Dr. Rafael Santonja (Spain), past President of the Olympic Weight Lifting Federation of Spain, and Professor Dr. Eduardo H. De Rose (Brazil), of the International Olympic Medical Commission.